Evolution of Treatments of Prostate Cancer: From Biology to Current Advanced Technologies

Evolution of Treatments of Prostate Cancer: From Biology to Current Advanced Technologies

Guest Editor

Fernando Munoz

MDPI

Basel • Beijing • Wuhan • Barcelona • Belgrade • Novi Sad • Cluj • Manchester

Guest Editor
Fernando Munoz
Radiation Oncology Department
'Umberto Parini' Regional Hospital
Aosta
Italy

Editorial Office
MDPI AG
Grosspeteranlage 5
4052 Basel, Switzerland

This is a reprint of the Special Issue, published open access by the journal *Current Oncology* (ISSN 1718-7729), freely accessible at: https://www.mdpi.com/journal/curroncol/special_issues/7L530CIA41.

For citation purposes, cite each article independently as indicated on the article page online and as indicated below:

Lastname, A.A.; Lastname, B.B. Article Title. *Journal Name* **Year**, *Volume Number*, Page Range.

ISBN 978-3-7258-6065-4 (Hbk)
ISBN 978-3-7258-6066-1 (PDF)
https://doi.org/10.3390/books978-3-7258-6066-1

Contents

Current Oncology

MDPI

Article

Can Deep Learning-Based Auto-Contouring Software Achieve Accurate Pelvic Volume Delineation in Volumetric Image-Guided Radiotherapy for Prostate Cancer? A Preliminary Multicentric Analysis

Cristiano Grossi [1], Fernando Munoz [2,*], Ilaria Bonavero [2], Eulalie Joelle Tondji Ngassam [1], Elisabetta Garibaldi [2], Claudia Airaldi [3], Elena Celia [2], Daniela Nassisi [3], Andrea Brignoli [2], Elisabetta Trino [3], Lavinia Bianco [3], Silvia Leardi [3], Diego Bongiovanni [3], Chiara Valero [4] and Maria Grazia Ruo Redda [5]

1 Department of Oncology, University of Turin School of Medicine, 10126 Turin, Italy; cristiano.grossi93@gmail.com (C.G.); eulaliejoelle.tondjingassam@unito.it (E.J.T.N.)
2 Department of Radiation Oncology, Umberto Parini Hospital, 11100 Aosta, Italy; ibonavero@ausl.vda.it (I.B.); egaribaldi@ausl.vda.it (E.G.); ecelia@ausl.vda.it (E.C.); abrignoli@ausl.vda.it (A.B.)
3 Department of Radiation Oncology, Mauriziano Umberto I Hospital, 10128 Turin, Italy; cairaldi@mauriziano.it (C.A.); dnassisi@mauriziano.it (D.N.); etrino@mauriziano.it (E.T.); lvbianco@mauriziano.it (L.B.); sleardi@mauriziano.it (S.L.); dott.diegobongiovanni@gmail.com (D.B.)
4 Department of Medical Physics, Mauriziano Umberto I Hospital, 10128 Turin, Italy; cvalero@mauriziano.it
5 Department Oncology, University of Turin School of Medicine, Mauriziano Umberto I Hospital, 10128 Turin, Italy; mariagrazia.ruoredda@unito.it
* Correspondence: fmunoz@ausl.vda.it

Abstract: Background: Radiotherapy (RT) is a mainstay treatment for prostate cancer (PC). Accurate delineation of organs at risk (OARs) is crucial for optimizing the therapeutic window by minimizing side effects. Manual segmentation is time-consuming and prone to inter-operator variability. This study investigates the performance of Limbus® Contour® (LC), a deep learning-based auto-contouring software, in delineating pelvic structures in PC patients. Methods: We evaluated LC's performance on key structures (bowel bag, bladder, rectum, sigmoid colon, and pelvic lymph nodes) in 52 patients. We compared auto-contoured structures with those manually delineated by radiation oncologists using different metrics. Results: LC achieved good agreement for the bladder (median Dice: 0.95) and rectum (median Dice: 0.83). However, limitations were observed for the bowel bag (median Dice: 0.64) and sigmoid colon (median Dice: 0.6), with inclusion of irrelevant structures. While the median Dice for pelvic lymph nodes was acceptable (0.73), the software lacked sub-regional differentiation, limiting its applicability in certain other oncologic settings. Conclusions: LC shows promise for automating OAR delineation in prostate radiotherapy, particularly for the bladder and rectum. Improvements are needed for bowel bag, sigmoid colon, and lymph node sub-regionalization. Further validation with a broader and larger patient cohort is recommended to assess generalizability.

Keywords: auto-contouring; organs at risk; deep learning; segmentation; prostate cancer; pelvic lymph nodes; Limbus® Contour

1. Introduction

Prostate cancer is the most common malignancy in the male population and consumes a significant number of resources in Radiation Oncology departments [1–3]. In Italy, prostate cancer accounts for over 20% of all cancers diagnosed in men over the age of 50. In

2022, there were approximately 40,500 new cases, while in 2023, the number increased to 41,100 and in 2024 it was 40,192. In total, 8200 men died because of prostate cancer in Italy in 2022 [4].

The treatment of prostate cancer must be personalized, considering the stage and aggressiveness of the disease, as well as the patient's life expectancy and the presence of any comorbidities that may increase the risk of mortality compared to the prostate cancer itself.

Radiotherapy (RT) is a therapeutic option for the treatment of prostate cancer with curative intent [5–12]. Equally radical prostatectomy (RP), involving surgical removal of the prostate, vas deferens, and seminal vesicles (with or without lymphadenectomy), is a common treatment for prostate cancer. However, even after RP, biochemical recurrence of disease (BCR) occurs in 27–53% of patients [13,14]. Adjuvant radiotherapy (ART) following RP has demonstrated a 50% reduction in BCR risk for patients with high-risk features [15–17]. A recent large retrospective study further emphasizes the benefit of ART in patients with positive lymph nodes (pN1), a high Gleason score (pathological GS 8–10), and extra prostatic extension (pT3/pT4), showing a reduction in all-cause mortality rates [18]. The salvage setting after RP, where cancer recurs, has become a crucial area of research. The ARTISTIC meta-analysis, encompassing trials like RADICALS-RT, TROG 08.03/ANZUP RAVES, and GETUG-AFU 17, supports the PSA-based approach and the role of salvage radiotherapy (SRT) in patients who were previously considered candidates for ART [19–22]. The RTOG 0534 trial showed a marginal benefit of prophylactic pelvic nodal irradiation (PNRT or ENRT) [23]. Consequently, RT plays an essential role in prostate cancer management in both radical and salvage setting by delivering a targeted high dose to eradicate cancerous cells while minimizing harm to surrounding healthy tissues. This delicate balance is crucial for mitigating both short- and long-term side effects. However, a major bottleneck in the treatment planning process is the manual segmentation of target volumes and organs at risk (OARs) on Computed Tomography (CT) scans [24]. Historically, manual segmentation of structures on 3D anatomical images, typically CT scans, has been performed by clinical experts. While this ensures expert review, it is also a very time-consuming process. Literature reports mean manual segmentation times for head and neck cases ranging significantly, from 28.5 min up to 3 h, depending on the specific structures being delineated. This time-intensive nature, coupled with the inherent susceptibility of manual segmentation to inter- and intra-observer variability, has driven the increasing adoption of automatic techniques over the past decade [25].

While manual contouring of organs at risk (OARs) and clinical target volumes (CTVs) is an essential component of radiotherapy (RT) planning, its time-consuming nature and reliance on staff availability contribute substantially to RT treatment planning lead times [26].

Artificial Intelligence (AI) can provide a powerful contribution to a lot of human-dependent steps in RT, considering that human participation is a principal uncertainty source, potentially impacting on the efficacy of treatments. In particular, the main fields of applications of AI in RT are the following:

- Lesion and OAR contouring, with data derived from fusions of multimodal imaging: The accuracy of auto-segmentation is higher for structures that have a high contrast against their surrounding tissues (lung, eye, bladder), while it is lower in the case of OARs with small volumes and fuzzy boundaries (optic chiasma). In clinical practice, manual checking is necessary, with a consideration of the different reference guidelines of different institutions.
- Treatment Planning: AI can help in augmenting dose map prediction (Dose Volume Histograms (DVHs) and voxel-based dose prediction) and in supervising and guiding the optimization process, which usually requires sequential modifications of parameters such as target coverage, OAR constraints and their priorities, selecting the ones

that need an update and also allowing for procedures of replanning and adaptive RT to be completed more quickly.

- Patient- and machine-specific quality assurance: The purpose of this is to ensure consistency between the medical prescription and its delivery, reducing the workload involved in measuring and analyzing doses using a phantom and in the assessment of the performances of all devices involved in RT. AI algorithms can also help in relating the spatial dose to RT outcomes, consenting prognosis predictions and prediction of the risk of side effects.

A major limitation in the use of AI in RT practice is the lack of regulation, because these systems do not have 100% accuracy, so human surveillance is essential. Furthermore, the use of AI could lead to young radiation oncologists dealing with matters beyond their level of expertise, since they have to face problems and devise solutions, particularly in checking results. This could cause issues in the advancements made within the discipline [27].

A thorough comprehension of these technologies is essential to warranting the optimal use of these tools. Advanced AI techniques, like Convolutional Neural Networks (CNNs) with high-performance predictions for complex problems, lead to the so-called "black box" problem: a lack of transparency and knowledge about the functioning of the machine learning models. This cultural barrier can dampen the faith in AI solutions held by health professionals. A technology known as Explainable AI (XAI) has the objective of clarifying how predictions are made, offering an insight into the internal mechanisms of these algorithms [28].

There is a real need for effective Uncertainty Quantification (UQ) methods, which could incentivize clinicians' confidence in and integration of AI models into clinical practice. UQ methods, both for epistemic and aleatoric uncertainties, are well established in computer science and are useful for the characterization of the limits of AI tools, but they are only in the early stages in their applications in healthcare. In the auto-segmentation field, methods such as conformal prediction can help in flagging cases with a low probability of correct segmentation and which need further human intervention [29].

Among the automated approaches, atlas-based segmentation methods have gained popularity in commercial systems. These methods typically involve selecting one or more pre-segmented atlases and deforming them to match the patient's anatomy to generate contours. Various methods exist for selecting the best atlas or combination of atlases [25].

Studies have evaluated atlas-based auto-segmentation for different anatomical sites and structures, including head and neck OARs and prostate OARs. For example, research has assessed atlas-based auto-segmentation tools for the head and neck OARs, pre-clinically and clinically validating them for multiple target volumes and normal tissues like swallowing and mastication structures [30].

More recently, advances in machine learning, particularly deep learning, have led to the development of sophisticated automated segmentation and planning tools [26,30–34].

Deep learning algorithms, such as CNNs and Fully Convolutional Networks (FCNs), have shown promise in segmenting anatomical structures [30].

Examples include deep learning for the clinically applicable segmentation of head and neck anatomy and the automated CT segmentation of prostate cancer anatomy [31,35].

Traditionally, the auto-segmentation approach was based on intensity analysis (based on differences in imaging intensity among different tissues), shape modeling (based on the typical anatomical aspect of the structures of interest), and atlas-based techniques (based on a database of previously delineated structures), derived from retrospective peer reviewed treatment contours. They required substantial manual editing. The advent of deep learning models, especially CNNs, has led to a paradigm shift in auto-segmentation approaches. Indeed, they can handle a wider variety of complex anatomical structures; in particular,

CNNs can extract hierarchical features from medical images through layers of learned convolutional filters [36].

Machine learning and AI applications are rapidly finding their way into the radiotherapy workflow.

Auto-segmentation solutions, particularly those leveraging deep learning, are being actively explored to alleviate these burdens, with the latter demonstrating improved accuracy over atlas-based techniques [31]. Despite this potential, the translation of deep learning-based auto-segmentation into routine clinical practice has been slow [3]. This delay in its adoption is likely associated with the current lack of comprehensive knowledge and standardized guidelines for the effective commissioning and implementation of these machine learning tools [3,32]. Moreover, this time-consuming and subjective task can lead to both inter and intra-variability between healthcare professionals.

Radici et al. reported time savings across multiple sites using Limbus Contour®, with the maximum advantages seen in head and neck cancer (65%-time savings), though time reductions for prostate (44%), breast (25%), and rectum (38%) have also been reported [37].

The recent emergence of AI used in medicine has also led to innovations in radiation oncology, offering significant advancements in treatment precision and workflow [38]. Recent advancements in AI have led to the development of auto-segmentation algorithms capable of delineating anatomical structures with a precision that rivals the expertise of human radiation oncologists. Watkins et al. explored the efficiency gains achievable with unedited AI-generated contours in total marrow irradiation, highlighting the potential of AI to achieve a 100% improvement in efficiency compared to traditional manual methods [39]. Another study reported that deep learning-based auto-segmentation reduces contouring time and improves clinical workflow efficiency in the treatment of cervical cancer [40]. A study focusing on the auto-segmentation of target volumes and OARs in pediatric cancer patients emphasized the importance of both accuracy and time efficiency in this vulnerable group. The study highlighted the potential of AI to strike a delicate balance between effective treatment and the preservation of normal tissue, which is crucial for minimizing potential growth-related complications in young patients [41]. Prior research suggests that AI can perform radiation contouring with a precision comparable to, if not exceeding, that of human oncologists. However, the strongest evidence of AI's efficacy lies in its ability to replicate the nuanced expertise of human practitioners. In the AI conference co-hosted by the Embassy of the Republic of Korea to the UAE, the Department of Health Abu Dhabi, and G42 Healthcare, comparative analysis was conducted, during which human radiation oncologists and the AI software Limbus® AI were tasked with contouring the axilla and internal mammary nodal chain from CT scans of a post-lumpectomy breast cancer patient. Only a small proportion of healthcare professionals and AI experts could correctly identify the AI-generated contour [42].

Auto-segmentation, facilitated by AI, holds promise for streamlining the manual contouring process. Studies suggest that AI can not only enhance efficiency but also reduce discrepancies arising from clinician interpretations [24,31]. Deep learning-based auto-segmented contours (DCs) have demonstrated remarkable accuracy, closely matching that of manual contours and surpassing that of traditional atlas-based methods [24,43] (Figure 1).

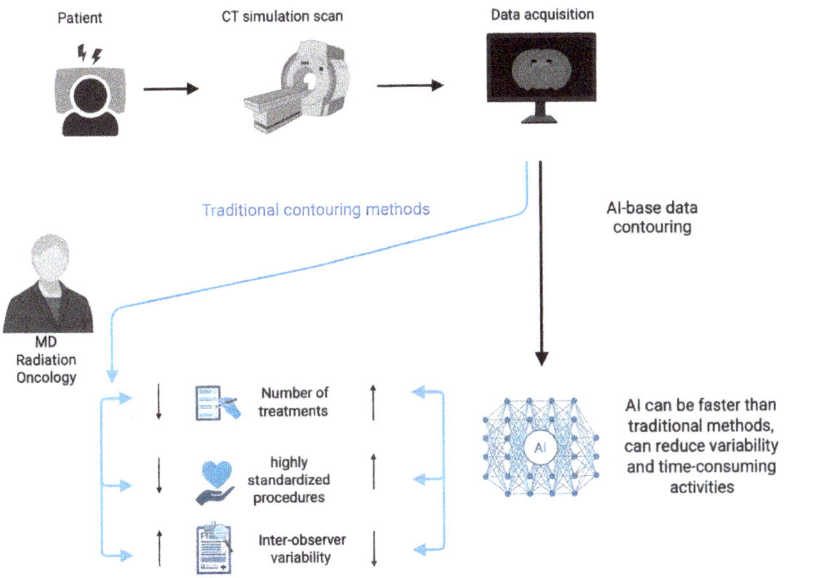

Figure 1. Comparison between traditional contouring methods used in radiation oncology and AI-based data contouring. Created in BioRender. Cristiano Grossi. (2025) https://app.biorender.com/illustrations/681bc74040787bb5138b50f9.

Despite the promising capabilities of AI-powered contouring, widespread clinical adoption remains limited [32]. Wong et al. reported the impact of DC models in the clinical workflow at two centers; in a previous study, they also conducted a comparison between DC and multiple radiation oncologists for central nervous system (CNS), head and neck (H&N), and prostate OARs and CTVs [24].

Further research is necessary to address the variability observed in the quality of DC models [33,44]. Rigorous studies are crucial to verify the reliability of specific models before their full integration into routine clinical practice [34]. This focus on robust validation will ensure the safe and effective implementation of AI in radiation oncology.

Seeking to streamline the radiotherapy workflow, in our institution, we investigated the clinical implementation of a commercial deep learning-based auto-contouring software. Wong et al. in 2020 reported on investigated CTVs in HN cancer and prostate gland cancer, but nonpelvic CTVs were included in their analysis [24].

Ethical concerns need to be considered in the development phase of AI tools. Ethical considerations in AI applications in healthcare call attention to issues such as security and privacy, the evaluation of AI models' reliability, the appropriate settings of applications of AI models, the allocation of responsibilities and the need for human monitoring of the results obtained with AI processes. Instruments for systematic ethical assessments of generative AI in healthcare have been developed, such as the TREGAI checklist, based on nine generally recognized ethical principles [45].

In this study, we aimed to assess the software's impact on contouring key pelvic structures, especially major pelvic lymph nodes, but also including the bowel, bladder, rectum, and sigmoid colon, within a homogeneous population with a diagnosis of PC. This study represents the first evaluation of major pelvic lymph node contouring, and may act as a valuable reference for other oncological diseases, including rectal cancer, anal canal cancer, and gynecological malignancies.

2. Materials and Methods

To streamline the radiotherapy workflow at our institutions, we investigated the clinical implementation of Limbus Contour software (Limbus AI Inc., Regina, SK, Canada, version 1.7.1) [46]. This study assessed the software's impact on the contouring of key pelvic structures, including the bowel, the bladder, the rectum, the sigmoid colon, and major pelvic lymph nodes.

For this study, we investigated the consistency and the geometric reliability of LC in patients with PC and pelvic lymph node involvement. Our analysis deliberately excluded the prostate gland, because previous authors previously demonstrated the accuracy of this method for delineating the whole prostate gland [47]. Our focus was on structures located outside the prostate gland.

We chose to evaluate pelvic structures due to their high inter-patient variability. This characteristic makes them a good target for testing the software's robustness in handling anatomical variations. Traditional segmentation methods, like atlas-based approaches, rely on pre-segmented image databases, which often require significant editing [25,43]. AI-powered contouring tools, like Limbus Contour, aim to overcome these limitations by offering quicker and more accurate delineations of target volumes and OARs. This has the potential to significantly improve patient outcomes through more precise radiation delivery [37].

We retrospectively analyzed data from 52 patients, treated at Mauriziano Umberto I Hospital, Turin, and "Umberto Parini" Hospital, Aosta, Italy, diagnosed with PC, comprising 40 patients with locally advanced PC and 12 patients with recurrent PC, treated between 2018 and 2024. All patients received either radical radiotherapy or adjuvant radiotherapy using the Volumetric Modulated Arc Therapy-Image Guided Radiotherapy (VMAT-IGRT) technique. All patients provided written informed consent approved by our Internal Institutional Review Board.

2.1. Software Description

In this study, we employed LC version 1.7.1, a commercially available auto-contouring software powered by deep learning algorithms. This advanced tool utilizes deep CNNs, with each anatomical structure being assigned a dedicated model specifically tailored for its unique features. These models are based on the widely adopted U-net architecture, a neural network design recognized for its effectiveness in biomedical image segmentation tasks [30,48,49].

The training process for LC models draws from an extensive and diverse array of imaging datasets. These include both publicly accessible datasets and proprietary collections obtained through collaborations with a range of medical institutions. Together, these sources form a robust and heterogeneous foundation for training the models, enhancing their generalizability and performance across different patient populations and imaging conditions [50–59]. The number of scans used to train each model typically ranges from several hundred to several thousand, ensuring that each model is supported by a substantial volume of learning data, which contributes to its accuracy and reliability.

To maintain high standards of performance and clinical relevance, Limbus AI implements a stringent dual-phase validation strategy. The first phase is an internal validation, where the software's auto-generated contours are systematically compared against expert-drawn annotations on a designated test dataset. This process provides an initial benchmark of the model's precision and segmentation accuracy. The second phase involves external validation through peer-reviewed publications, where independent studies assess both the qualitative and quantitative performance of the models. These studies also explore the software's ability to enhance and expedite clinical workflows, thereby supporting its utility in real-world radiotherapy planning scenarios [24,50].

2.2. Contouring Process and Data Analysis

In this study, we assessed the level of concordance between organ delineations automatically generated by the Limbus AI software and those manually contoured by three experienced radiation oncologists using the RayStation System (RaySearch Laboratories, Stockolm, Sweden) as the treatment planning system (TPS), with the latest version available in 2024. The treatment plans and contours from our institutions were retrieved for analysis. The anatomical structures selected for delineation and analysis included key OARs and target volumes relevant to pelvic radiotherapy, specifically the bowel bag, bladder, rectum, and sigmoid colon, as well as the pelvic lymph nodes, which were contoured as part of the CTV. These structures were chosen due to their clinical importance in treatment planning and the potential variability in manual contouring. For each patient case, a duplicate set of the original manually defined structures was created within the Limbus software. These auto-generated contours were designed to mirror the original anatomical regions but were automatically labeled with a "Limbus" suffix. This labeling strategy was employed to clearly distinguish between the auto-contoured structures and those manually delineated by the radiation oncologists, ensuring clarity during subsequent analyses.

These new Regions of Interest (ROIs) were then exported back to RayStation for analysis using custom Python scripting (version 3.12) in terms of the following metrics:

1. Volume: The absolute volume of each ROI expressed in cubic centimeters (cc).
2. Dice Coefficient (DC): A measure of conformity, reflecting the spatial overlap between two delineated volumes. A value of 1 indicates perfect overlap.
3. Precision: The proportion of voxels identified by Limbus that truly belong to the OAR, reflecting the accuracy of inclusion. A value of 1 indicates only true positives (with no irrelevant structures included).
4. Sensitivity: The proportion of voxels in the true OAR that are correctly identified by Limbus, reflecting the completeness of delineation. A value of 1 indicates all true positives (no missed voxels).
5. Specificity: The proportion of voxels outside the true OAR that are correctly excluded by Limbus, reflecting the ability to avoid irrelevant structures. A value of 1 indicates only true negatives (with no false positives included).
6. Mean Distance to Agreement (Mean DA): The average distance between the surfaces of structures identified in both delineations and those identified by only one delineation. A value of 0 indicates perfect agreement in surface location.
7. Maximum Distance to Agreement (Max DA): The largest distance between any corresponding surface points in the two delineations. A value of 0 indicates perfect spatial overlap.

The following sections will provide detailed explanations of each metric (precision, sensitivity, specificity, Mean DA, and Max DA) in the context of organ delineation and their clinical significance.

3. Results

Fifty-two patients were included in this retrospective analysis. Table 1 summarizes the dosimetric evaluation of organ delineation using all metrics listed previously.

Table 1. The median average of all dosimetric data evaluated for each structure.

	CTV	Bowel	Bladder	Rectum	Sigmoid
Diff. Vol (cc)	−56.82 (−205.96; 185.94)	−417.25 (−1500.57; 5168)	−0.09 (−22.27; 14.58)	3.05 (−18.91; 23.73)	−13.68 (−198.91; 82.34)
Dice	0.73 (0.53; 0.84)	0.62 (0.36; 1)	0.97 (0.77; 1)	0.87 (0.57; 1)	0.60 (0.2; 1)
Precision	0.58 (0.36; 0.73)	0.45 (0.22; 1)	0.94 (0.63; 1)	0.76 (0.4; 1)	0.44 (0.11; 1)
Sensitivity	0.79 (0.57; 0.97)	0.65 (0.24; 1)	0.97 (0.76; 1)	0.86 (0.61; 1)	0.85 (0.22; 1)
Specificity	0.65 (−0.2; 0.96)	0.83 (−1.08; 1)	0.98 (0.72; 1)	0.91 (0.09; 1)	0.41 (−6.93; 1)
Mean DA	0.39 (0.18; 0.97)	1.2 (0.01; 3.98)	0.07 (0; 0.35)	0.15 (0; 1)	0.73 (0; 3.43)
Max DA	3.25 (1.76; 6.65)	8.39 (0.02; 16.51)	0.66 (0.01; 2.26)	1.3 (0.01; 5.52)	5.44 (0.01; 17.09)

CTV achieved good agreement with clinician contours, with a median Dice of 0.73 and a median volume difference of −56.82 cc. However, the model's precision for CTV segmentation was lower (0.58), indicating a higher rate of false positives. In some cases, non-target structures like the bowel were included in the segmentation. The sensitivity was better than specificity (0.79 and 0.65, respectively). These findings suggest that, while the model can accurately delineate the CTV, in some cases, false structures were included in CTV, so further refinement is necessary to improve the precision of segmenting this structure. In contrast, delineation of the bowel bag using LC resulted in a lower median Dice coefficient (0.60) and a larger median volume difference −417.25 cc. This discrepancy likely arises from the excessively large LC margins incorporating the neighboring structures within the bag, as reflected by the lower precision (0.45) value for the bowel bag segmentation. Specificity reached an unexpectedly high value (0.83).

Bladder delineation achieved excellent agreement, with the highest median Dice (0.97) among the OARs evaluated (Figure 2). Volume differences were also minimal (median: −0.09 cc). A similarly excellent result was also obtained for precision, specificity, and sensitivity (0.94, 0.97, and 0.98, respectively). The mean DA achieved was 0.07, with a maximum DA of 0.66.

Similarly to the outcomes for the bowel bag segmentation, sigmoid delineation using LC proved challenging. The median Dice value for the sigmoid was 0.6, and the median volume difference was −13.68 cc. Precision was confirmed to be very poor, at 0.44, the worst of all analyzed structures. Similarly, the specificity was 0.41. We frequently observed inconsistencies between the LC-defined cranial margin of the sigmoid and the clinician's delineation. In some cases, a gap existed between the sigmoid and the rectal Limbus Contour. In contrast, the rectum exhibited good agreement with a median Dice value of 0.76 and a negligible median volume difference, 3.05 cc. The precision value was 0.76, and the sensitivity was 0.86; therefore, LC did not miss many voxels.

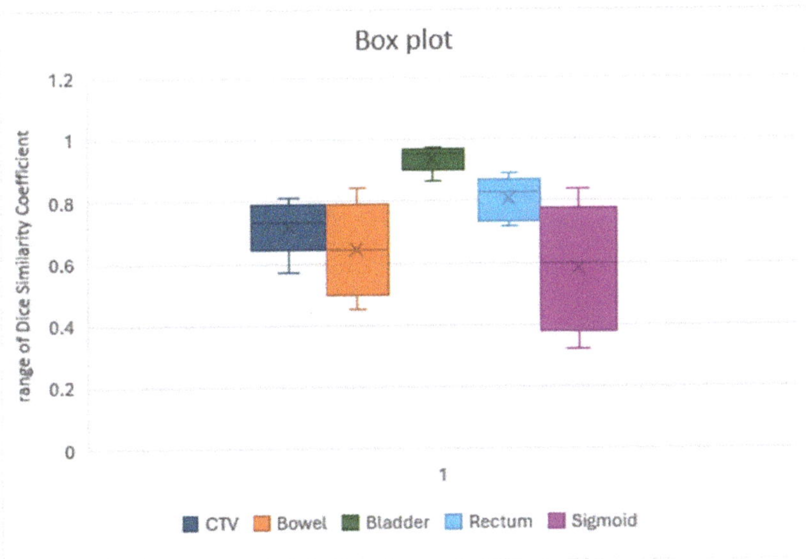

Figure 2. Variability range of Dice distribution for the CTV and OARs analyzed. The bladder achieved the best results, with the least differences, while the sigmoid had the worst results, with wide variability and the lowest median Dice. Similar results were obtained with the bowel. The rectum had excellent results. The CTV reached an acceptable value for a short while.

4. Discussion

The present study investigated the clinical implementation of a commercial deep learning-based auto-contouring software (Limbus Contour, LC, version 1.8) for PC patients with pelvic lymph node involvement in a radiation therapy workflow.

The primary aim was to evaluate the software's impact on the contouring of key pelvic structures, with a particular focus on major pelvic lymph nodes, alongside the bowel bag, bladder, rectum, and sigmoid colon (Figure 3).

To the best of our knowledge, this research represents the first evaluation of major pelvic lymph node contouring using an auto-contouring software, acting as a potentially valuable reference for other pelvic malignancies.

Previous studies have extensively evaluated the performance of auto-segmentation software, including deep learning models, for commonly contoured organs-at-risk (OARs) such as the bladder, rectum, and prostate, often demonstrating excellent results [37,60,61].

Van Dijk et al. classified vDSC (volumetric Dice similarity coefficient) scores into good (vDSC > 0.8), good–intermediate (0.7 < vDSC < 0.8), intermediate (0.6 < vDSC < 0.7), intermediate–poor (0.5 < vDSC < 0.6), and poor (vDSC < 0.5) [62]. However, it is important to remember that vDSC scores are relative; a score of 0.8 signifies high accuracy for small organs like optic nerves but indicates lower accuracy for larger structures such as the bowel or lungs. While we observed a good median Dice coefficient for the CTV (0.73), with the value generally considered clinically acceptable being around 0.72, according to previous studies [61], a major limitation exists. Unlike head and neck applications where lymph node sub-regions are identified and contoured separately, LC does not generate different structures for iliac, obturator, presacral, or inguinal lymph nodes and does not contour inguinal or lombo-aortic lymph nodes. This hinders its applicability in gynecological and gastrointestinal cancers, in which these important lymph node stations are absent. However, these settings are beyond the scope of our investigation.

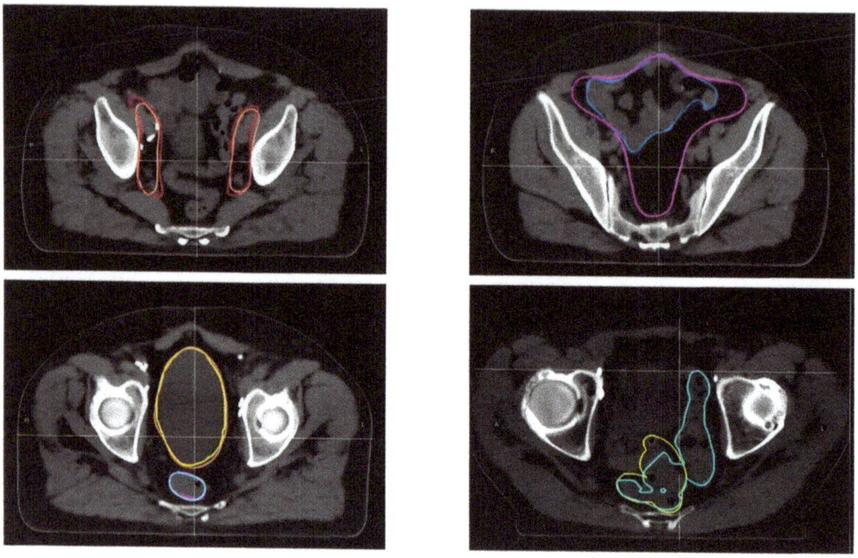

Figure 3. Orange CTV made by radiation oncologists, Red CTV made by Limbus; Blue Bowel made by radiation oncologists, Purple Bowel made by Limbus; Yellow Bladder made by radiation oncologists, Orange Bladder made by Limbus; Pink Rectum made by radiation oncologists, Light blue Rectum made by Limbus; Olive sigmoid made by radiation oncologists, Turquoise sigmoid made by Limbus. Orange line: CTV contoured by radiation oncologists. Red line: CTV contoured by LC. Blue bowel: bowel contoured by radiation oncologists. Purple bowel: bowel contoured by LC. Yellow bladder: contoured by radiation oncologists. Orange bladder: contoured by LC. Pink rectum: contoured by radiation oncologists. Light blue rectum: contoured by LC. Olive sigmoid: contoured by radiation oncologists. Turquoise sigmoid: contoured by LC.

Despite the strong performance of AI on many OARs, it is crucial to note that certain structures or specific regions often require significant manual editing. In a study by Cha et al. focusing on prostate Stereotactic Body Radiation Therapy (SBRT), 33% of the auto-contours required major, clinically significant edits based on physician surveys. While OARs generally required minimal to moderate changes, structures like the CTV in the pelvic region (specifically the prostate and seminal vesicles in the study mentioned) and the penile bulb had a greater necessity for significant modification [31].

Wong et al., evaluating deep learning-based auto-contours, reported that for bladder and rectum OARs, the average editing scores were 2 or less on a five-point scale (where 1 means minimal editing) [24].

Similarly, Zabel et al. compared manual contouring (MANpreRO) with atlas-based (ATLASpreRO) and deep learning-based (DEEPpreRO, using Limbus Contour) auto-contouring for the bladder and rectum in prostate cancer patients. Their findings indicated that DEEPpreRO contours showed greater geometric similarity to manual contours, with significantly higher DSC values and a lower Mean Surface Distance (MSS) for both structures [60].

Radici et al., using Limbus Contour for various sites, reported an average DSC of 0.72 across all analyzed structures [37].

The performance of LC varied across the different OARs, as can be seen in Figure 2. Bladder delineation achieved excellent agreement, with a high median Dice coefficient (0.97) and good precision (0.94), specificity (0.97), and sensitivity (0.98). This aligns with previous findings in several studies [60,63]; Kim et al. reported a lower Dice value, but they tested LC version 1.5 and 1.6 only on 10 pelvic patients [64]. In an earlier atlas-based study carried out in 2016, Wong et al. [65] reported median DSC values of 0.90 for the bladder, 0.77 for the rectum, and 0.84 for the prostate with the recommended settings. These values generally support the potential of deep learning to achieve high geometric similarity for common pelvic OARs.

However, bowel delineation presented challenges. The median Dice coefficient (0.62) was lower than that for the bladder, and the precision (0.45) was particularly poor, indicating the inclusion of irrelevant structures. This finding aligns with Radici et al. [37], who reported discrepancies between manual and automatic bowel segmentation. Doolan et al. analyzed only 20 prostate patients with five commercial AI auto-segmentation devices and reported a very low dice value (vDSC 0.59−0.76) for the bowels, but they did not test LC [66].

LC offers the opportunity to choose between single loops or whole-bowel delineation. In our study, whole-bowel volumes were significantly larger than manually contoured ones, potentially impacting treatment planning.

Although LC's performance was evaluated for abdominal OARs in a recent study, the bowel was not included in our analysis [67].

Similar results were observed for the sigmoid. While the median Dice coefficient (0.6) suggests some overlap, the low precision (0.44) indicates the frequent inclusion of non-sigmoid structures. In further detail, discrepancies in manual and LC delineation of the rectosigmoid junction were frequently observed.

LC's capabilities regarding rectum contouring were totally different. Our study reported a Dice coefficient of 0.87a, value close to that (0.86) reported in previous research by Zabel et al. [60] and Oktay et al. (0.90) [63], indicating good overlap with manual contours. However, our study suggests that LC may exhibit greater difficulty with sigmoid contouring compared to contouring of the rectum, a limitation seen with many other AI auto-segmentation softwares [66]. This aligns with our findings of a lower Dice coefficient and lower precision for the sigmoid.

Despite the difficulties in precisely quantifying the time savings, perceived utility and observed improvements in workflow efficiency are frequently reported. Zabel et al. found that deep learning auto-contouring (using Limbus Contour) for the bladder and rectum significantly reduced the initial contour generation time (1.4 min for DEEP vs. 10.9 min for manual) without significantly increasing the time required for physician editing compared to manual methods (4.7 min for DEEP editing vs. 4.1 min for manual editing) [61].

This study has limitations, including its retrospective design and limited sample size. Further research with a larger and more diverse patient population is necessary for generalizability. Future studies should investigate the potential of AI algorithms to accurately delineate not only pelvic lymph nodes in various cancer types, but also the bowel and sigmoid. This could significantly improve the efficiency of radiotherapy planning and reduce the workload for radiation oncologists.

Another limitation is the lack of a dedicated dosimetric analysis to assess the impact of using auto-contours instead of manual contours in terms of DVH metrics.

The most recent version of LC, version 1.8, can contour new structures for example inguinal lymph nodes station, but it cannot contour other structures for example lombo-aortic lymph nodes yet. Furthermore, differentiation of pelvic lymph nodes (iliac, obturator, and presacral), such as those in the head and neck cancer setting, is not permitted.

Overall, this study provides valuable insights into the potential and limitations of using LC as a supporting instrument for pelvic structure delineation in radiotherapy. Accurate comparison with studies in the previously published literature is inherently difficult. This is due to variations in the definition of "gold-standard" manual contours, differences in arbitration and consensus-building processes, variations in the datasets used (including patient demographics, disease sites, stages, and tumor types), diverse scanning parameters and image devices, and different labeling protocols [30].

Quantifying time savings accurately in a real-world clinical setting remains challenging.

5. Conclusions

In conclusion, the findings from this study, supported by the growing body of evidence in existing research, demonstrate the capability of deep learning approaches to achieve high-quality auto-segmentation for radiotherapy, often reaching performance levels comparable to that of human experts for common OARs. The evaluation of Limbus Contour, particularly for pelvic structures, confirms its potential utility in the clinical workflow by reducing the initial contouring burden and providing suitable starting points for required edits. While significant progress has been made, particularly for well-defined OARs, challenges remain in achieving consistent accuracy for all structures and in precisely quantifying the impact on clinical workflow efficiency. Continued refinement of AI models, addressing areas of frequent editing, establishing clinical consensus on contouring protocols, and providing adequate training and robust QA frameworks are necessary steps to maximize the benefits of auto-segmentation in radiotherapy and improve consistency and safety in clinical practice. These challenges require further development and validation before AI's broader clinical adoption.

By overcoming these limitations and exploring LC's applicability across diverse cancer types, we can significantly improve the efficiency and precision of treatment planning in the future. Ultimately, this translates to better patient outcomes in cancer care. Continued advancements in AI-driven technologies hold immense potential for optimizing radiotherapy.

Author Contributions: C.G. was responsible for conceptualization, methodology, and writing—original draft preparation. C.G. also contributed to writing—review and editing. I.B. contributed to acquisition of data, resources, writing—original draft preparation, and writing—review and editing. E.J.T.N. contributed to conceptualization, data curation, formal analysis, and visualization. C.A., E.T. and E.G. were involved in investigation and resource acquisition. E.C. and A.B. contributed to the acquisition of data and to the investigation. D.N., L.B., S.L. and D.B. provided supervision and contributed to writing—review and editing. C.V. contributed to methodology, software, and data curation. Finally, M.G.R.R. and F.M. contributed to writing—review and editing, project administration, and validation. All authors have read and agreed to the published version of the manuscript.

Funding: This research received no external funding.

Institutional Review Board Statement: All procedures performed in our study involving human participants were in accordance with the ethical standards of the institutional and/or national research committee, and with the principles of the 1964 Declaration of Helsinki and its later amendments or comparable ethical standards. Ethical review and approval were waived for this study because the privacy of the patients was respected, with anonimization of their data and the retrospective nature of this analysis did not had an impact on the therapy administered to the patients.

Informed Consent Statement: Informed consent was obtained from all subjects involved in the study.

Data Availability Statement: The data presented in this study are available on request from the corresponding author.

Conflicts of Interest: The authors declare no conflicts of interest.

Abbreviations

The following abbreviations are used in this manuscript:

RT	Radiotherapy
PC	Prostate Cancer
OARs	Organs at risk
LC	Limbus contour
RP	Radical Prostatectomy
BCR	Biochemical Recurrence
ART	Adjuvant Radiotherapy
GS	Gleason Score
SRT	Salvage Radiotherapy
PNRT	Pelvic Nodal Radiotherapy
ENRT	Elective Nodal Radiotherapy
CT	Computed Tomography
CTV	Clinical target volume
AI	Artificial Intelligence
DVHs	Dose Volume Histograms
CNNs	Convolutional Neural Networks
XAI	Explainable AI
UQ	Uncertainty Quantification
FCNs	Fully Convolutional Networks
DCs	Deep Learning-Based Auto-Segmented Contours
CNS	Central Nervous System
H&N	Head and Neck
VMAT-IGRT	Volumetric Modulated Arc Therapy-Image Guided Radiotherapy
TPS	Treatment Planning System
ROIs	Regions Of Interest
cc	Cubic Centimeters
DC	Dice Coefficient
DA	Distance to Agreement
vDSC	Volumetric Dice Similarity Coefficient
SBRT	Stereotactic Body Radiation Therapy
DEEP	Deep learning auto contour

References

1. Siegel, R.L.; Miller, K.D.; Jemal, A. Cancer statistics, 2016. *CA Cancer J. Clin.* **2016**, *66*, 7–30. [CrossRef] [PubMed]
2. Ferlay, J.; Steliarova-Foucher, E.; Lortet-Tieulent, J.; Rosso, S.; Coebergh, J.W.W.; Comber, H.; Forman, D.; Bray, F. Cancer incidence and mortality patterns in Europe: Estimates for 40 countries in 2012. *Eur. J. Cancer* **2013**, *49*, 1374–1403. [CrossRef]
3. Arnold, M.; Karim-Kos, H.E.; Coebergh, J.W.; Byrnes, G.; Antilla, A.; Ferlay, J.; Renehan, A.G.; Forman, D.; Soerjomataram, I. Recent trends in incidence of five common cancers in 26 European countries since 1988: Analysis of the European Cancer Observatory. *Eur. J. Cancer* **2013**, *51*, 1164–1187. [CrossRef]
4. AIOM. I Numeri del Cancro in Italia. Available online: https://www.aiom.it/i-numeri-del-cancro-in-italia/ (accessed on 11 May 2025).
5. Greco, C.; Vazirani, A.A.; Pares, O.; Pimentel, N.; Louro, V.; Morales, J.; Nunes, B.; Vasconcelos, A.L.; Antunes, I.; Kociolek, J.; et al. The evolving role of external beam radiotherapy in localized prostate cancer. *Semin. Oncol.* **2019**, *46*, 246–253. [CrossRef] [PubMed]
6. Pollack, A.; Zagars, G.K. External beam radiotherapy dose response of prostate cancer. *Int. J. Radiat. Oncol. Biol. Phys.* **1997**, *39*, 1011–1018. [CrossRef]
7. Zelefsky, M.; Leibel, S.; Gaudin, P.; Kutcher, G.; Fleshner, N.; Venkatramen, E.S.; Reuter, V.; Fair, W.; Ling, C.C.; Fuks, Z. Dose escalation with three-dimensional conformal radiation therapy affects the outcome in prostate cancer. *Int. J. Radiat. Oncol. Biol. Phys.* **1998**, *41*, 491–500. [CrossRef] [PubMed]
8. Kuban, D.A.; Tucker, S.L.; Dong, L.; Starkschall, G.; Huang, E.H.; Cheung, M.R.; Lee, A.K.; Pollack, A. Long-Term Results of the M. D. Anderson Randomized Dose-Escalation Trial for Prostate Cancer. *Int. J. Radiat. Oncol. Biol. Phys.* **2007**, *70*, 67–74. [CrossRef]
9. Pasalic, D.; Kuban, D.A.; Allen, P.K.; Tang, C.; Mesko, S.M.; Grant, S.R.; Augustyn, A.A.; Frank, S.J.; Choi, S.; Hoffman, K.E.; et al. Dose Escalation for Prostate Adenocarcinoma: A Long-Term Update on the Outcomes of a Phase 3, Single Institution Randomized Clinical Trial. *Int. J. Radiat. Oncol. Biol. Phys.* **2019**, *104*, 790–797. [CrossRef]

10. Spratt, D.E.; Pei, X.; Yamada, J.; Kollmeier, M.A.; Cox, B.; Zelefsky, M.J. Long-term Survival and Toxicity in Patients Treated with High-Dose Intensity Modulated Radiation Therapy for Localized Prostate Cancer. *Int. J. Radiat. Oncol. Biol. Phys.* **2012**, *85*, 686–692. [CrossRef]
11. Heemsbergen, W.D.; Al-Mamgani, A.; Slot, A.; Dielwart, M.F.H.; Lebesque, J.V. Long-term results of the Dutch randomized prostate cancer trial: Impact of dose-escalation on local, biochemical, clinical failure, and survival. *Radiother. Oncol.* **2013**, *110*, 104–109. [CrossRef]
12. Dearnaley, D.P.; Jovic, G.; Syndikus, I.; Khoo, V.; Cowan, R.A.; Graham, J.D.; Aird, E.G.; Bottomley, D.; Huddart, R.A.; Jose, C.C.; et al. Escalated-dose versus control-dose conformal radiotherapy for prostate cancer: Long-term results from the MRC RT01 randomised controlled trial. *Lancet Oncol.* **2014**, *15*, 464–473. [CrossRef] [PubMed]
13. Van Den Broeck, T.; Van Den Bergh, R.C.N.; Briers, E.; Cornford, P.; Cumberbatch, M.; Tilki, D.; De Santis, M.; Fanti, S.; Fossati, N.; Gillessen, S.; et al. Biochemical Recurrence in Prostate Cancer: The European Association of Urology Prostate Cancer Guidelines Panel Recommendations. *Eur. Urol. Focus* **2019**, *6*, 231–234. [CrossRef]
14. Freedland, S.J.; Humphreys, E.B.; Mangold, L.A.; Eisenberger, M.; Dorey, F.J.; Walsh, P.C.; Partin, A.W. Death in Patients with Recurrent Prostate Cancer After Radical Prostatectomy: Prostate-Specific Antigen Doubling Time Subgroups and Their Associated Contributions to All-Cause Mortality. *J. Clin. Oncol.* **2007**, *25*, 1765–1771. [CrossRef]
15. Bolla, M.; Van Poppel, H.; Tombal, B.; Vekemans, K.; Da Pozzo, L.; De Reijke, T.M.; Verbaeys, A.; Bosset, J.-F.; Van Velthoven, R.; Colombel, M.; et al. Postoperative radiotherapy after radical prostatectomy for high-risk prostate cancer: Long-term results of a randomised controlled trial (EORTC trial 22911). *Lancet* **2012**, *380*, 2018–2027. [CrossRef]
16. Zimmermann, M.; Taussky, D.; Delouya, G.; Alenizi, A.M.; Zorn, K.C. Radiation therapy after radical prostatectomy: A single-centre radiation oncology experience in trends of referral and treatment practices. *Can. Urol. Assoc. J.* **2015**, *9*, 608. [CrossRef] [PubMed]
17. Wiegel, T.; Bottke, D.; Steiner, U.; Siegmann, A.; Golz, R.; Störkel, S.; Willich, N.; Semjonow, A.; Souchon, R.; Stöckle, M.; et al. Phase III Postoperative Adjuvant Radiotherapy After Radical Prostatectomy Compared with Radical Prostatectomy Alone in pT3 Prostate Cancer with Postoperative Undetectable Prostate-Specific Antigen: ARO 96-02/AUO AP 09/95. *J. Clin. Oncol.* **2009**, *27*, 2924–2930. [CrossRef] [PubMed]
18. Tilki, D.; Chen, M.-H.; Wu, J.; Huland, H.; Graefen, M.; Wiegel, T.; Böhmer, D.; Mohamad, O.; Cowan, J.E.; Feng, F.Y.; et al. Adjuvant Versus Early Salvage Radiation Therapy for Men at High Risk for Recurrence Following Radical Prostatectomy for Prostate Cancer and the Risk of Death. *J. Clin. Oncol.* **2021**, *39*, 2284–2293. [CrossRef] [PubMed]
19. Vale, C.L.; Fisher, D.; Kneebone, A.; Parker, C.; Pearse, M.; Richaud, P.; Sargos, P.; Sydes, M.R.; Brawley, C.; Brihoum, M.; et al. Adjuvant or early salvage radiotherapy for the treatment of localised and locally advanced prostate cancer: A prospectively planned systematic review and meta-analysis of aggregate data. *Lancet* **2020**, *396*, 1422–1431. [CrossRef]
20. Parker, C.; Sydes, M.R.; Catton, C.; Kynaston, H.; Logue, J.; Murphy, C.; Morgan, R.C.; Mellon, K.; Morash, C.; Parulekar, W.; et al. Radiotherapy and androgen deprivation in combination after local surgery (RADICALS): A new Medical Research Council/National Cancer Institute of Canada phase III trial of adjuvant treatment after radical prostatectomy. *BJU Int.* **2007**, *99*, 1376–1379. [CrossRef]
21. Pearse, M.; Fraser-Browne, C.; Davis, I.D.; Duchesne, G.M.; Fisher, R.; Frydenberg, M.; Haworth, A.; Jose, C.; Joseph, D.J.; Lim, T.S.; et al. A Phase III trial to investigate the timing of radiotherapy for prostate cancer with high-risk features: Background and rationale of the Radiotherapy—Adjuvant Versus Early Salvage (RAVES) trial. *BJU Int.* **2014**, *113*, 7–12. [CrossRef]
22. Sargos, P.; Chabaud, S.; Latorzeff, I.; Magné, N.; Benyoucef, A.; Supiot, S.; Pasquier, D.; Abdiche, M.S.; Gilliot, O.; Graff-Cailleaud, P.; et al. Adjuvant radiotherapy versus early salvage radiotherapy plus short-term androgen deprivation therapy in men with localised prostate cancer after radical prostatectomy (GETUG-AFU 17): A randomised, phase 3 trial. *Lancet Oncol.* **2020**, *21*, 1341–1352. [CrossRef]
23. Pollack, A.; Karrison, T.G.; Balogh, A.G.; Gomella, L.G.; Low, D.A.; Bruner, D.W.; Wefel, J.S.; Martin, A.-G.; Michalski, J.M.; Angyalfi, S.J.; et al. The addition of androgen deprivation therapy and pelvic lymph node treatment to prostate bed salvage radiotherapy (NRG Oncology/RTOG 0534 SPPORT): An international, multicentre, randomised phase 3 trial. *Lancet* **2022**, *399*, 1886–1901. [CrossRef] [PubMed]
24. Wong, J.; Fong, A.; McVicar, N.; Smith, S.; Giambattista, J.; Wells, D.; Kolbeck, C.; Giambattista, J.; Gondara, L.; Alexander, A. Comparing deep learning-based auto-segmentation of organs at risk and clinical target volumes to expert inter-observer variability in radiotherapy planning. *Radiother. Oncol.* **2019**, *144*, 152–158. [CrossRef] [PubMed]
25. Schipaanboord, B.; Boukerroui, D.; Peressutti, D.; Van Soest, J.; Lustberg, T.; Dekker, A.; Van Elmpt, W.; Gooding, M.J. An Evaluation of Atlas Selection Methods for Atlas-Based Automatic Segmentation in Radiotherapy Treatment Planning. *IEEE Trans. Med. Imaging* **2019**, *38*, 2654–2664. [CrossRef] [PubMed]
26. Wong, J.; Huang, V.; Wells, D.; Giambattista, J.; Giambattista, J.; Kolbeck, C.; Otto, K.; Saibishkumar, E.P.; Alexander, A. Implementation of deep learning-based auto-segmentation for radiotherapy planning structures: A workflow study at two cancer centers. *Radiat. Oncol.* **2021**, *16*, 101. [CrossRef]

27. Shan, G.; Yu, S.; Lai, Z.; Xuan, Z.; Zhang, J.; Wang, B.; Ge, Y. A Review of Artificial Intelligence Application for Radiotherapy. *Dose-Response* **2024**, *22*, 3687. [CrossRef]
28. Karako, K.; Tang, W. Applications of and issues with machine learning in medicine: Bridging the gap with explainable AI. *Biosci. Trends* **2024**, *18*, 497–504. [CrossRef]
29. Wahid, K.A.; Wahida, B.; Kaffey, Z.Y.; Farris, D.P.; Humbert-Vidan, L.; Moreno, A.C.; Rasmussend, M.; Rend, J.; Naserb, M.A.; Nethertone, T.J.; et al. Artificial Intelligence Uncertainty Quantification in Radiotherapy Applications—A Scoping Review. *Radiother. Oncol.* **2024**, *201*, 110542. [CrossRef]
30. Nikolov, S.; Blackwell, S.; Zverovitch, A.; Mendes, R.; Livne, M.; De Fauw, J.; Patel, Y.; Meyer, C.; Askham, H.; Romera-Paredes, B.; et al. Clinically Applicable Segmentation of Head and Neck Anatomy for Radiotherapy: Deep Learning Algorithm Development and Validation Study. *J. Med. Internet Res.* **2021**, *23*, e26151. [CrossRef]
31. Cha, E.; Elguindi, S.; Onochie, I.; Gorovets, D.; Deasy, J.O.; Zelefsky, M.; Gillespie, E.F. Clinical implementation of deep learning contour autosegmentation for prostate radiotherapy. *Radiother. Oncol.* **2021**, *159*, 1–7. [CrossRef]
32. Brouwer, C.L.; Dinkla, A.M.; Vandewinckele, L.; Crijns, W.; Claessens, M.; Verellen, D.; Van Elmpt, W. Machine learning applications in radiation oncology: Current use and needs to support clinical implementation. *Phys. Imaging Radiat. Oncol.* **2020**, *16*, 144–148. [CrossRef] [PubMed]
33. Jiang, J.; Hu, Y.-C.; Liu, C.-J.; Halpenny, D.; Hellmann, M.D.; Deasy, J.O.; Mageras, G.; Veeraraghavan, H. Multiple Resolution Residually Connected Feature Streams for Automatic Lung Tumor Segmentation from CT Images. *IEEE Trans. Med. Imaging* **2018**, *38*, 134–144. [CrossRef] [PubMed]
34. Vandewinckele, L.; Claessens, M.; Dinkla, A.; Brouwer, C.; Crijns, W.; Verellen, D.; Van Elmpt, W. Overview of artificial intelligence-based applications in radiotherapy: Recommendations for implementation and quality assurance. *Radiother. Oncol.* **2020**, *153*, 55–66. [CrossRef] [PubMed]
35. Savenije, M.H.F.; Maspero, M.; Sikkes, G.G.; van der Voort van Zyp, J.R.N.; Kotte, A.N.; Bol, G.H.; T van den Berg, C.A. Clinical implementation of MRI-based organs-at-risk autosegmentation with convolutional networks for prostate radiotherapy. *Radiat. Oncol.* **2020**, *15*, 104. [CrossRef] [PubMed]
36. Erdur, A.C.; Rusche, D.; Scholz, D.; Kiechle, J.; Fischer, S.; Llorián-Salvador, Ó.; Buchner, J.A.; Nguyen, M.Q.; Etzel, L.; Weidner, J.; et al. Deep learning for autosegmentation for radiotherapy treatment planning: State-of-the-art and novel perspectives. *Strahlenther. Onkol.* **2025**, *201*, 236–254. [CrossRef]
37. Radici, L.; Ferrario, S.; Borca, V.C.; Cante, D.; Paolini, M.; Piva, C.; Baratto, L.; Franco, P.; La Porta, M.R. Implementation of a Commercial Deep Learning-Based Auto Segmentation Software in Radiotherapy: Evaluation of Effectiveness and Impact on Workflow. *Life* **2022**, *12*, 2088. [CrossRef]
38. Bibault, J.-E.; Giraud, P.; Burgun, A. Big Data and machine learning in radiation oncology: State of the art and future prospects. *Cancer Lett.* **2016**, *382*, 110–117. [CrossRef]
39. Watkins, W.T.; Qing, K.; Han, C.; Hui, S.; Liu, A. Auto-segmentation for total marrow irradiation. *Front. Oncol.* **2022**, *12*, 970425. [CrossRef]
40. Ma, C.Y.; Zhou, J.Y.; Xu, X.T.; Guo, J.; Han, M.F.; Gao, Y.Z.; Du, H.; Stahl, J.N.; Maltz, J.S. Deep learning-based auto-segmentation of clinical target volumes for radiotherapy treatment of cervical cancer. *J. Appl. Clin. Med. Phys.* **2022**, *23*, e13470. [CrossRef]
41. Qiu, W.; Zhang, W.; Ma, X.; Kong, Y.; Shi, P.; Fu, M.; Wang, D.; Hu, M.; Zhou, X.; Dong, Q.; et al. Auto-segmentation of important centers of growth in the pediatric skeleton to consider during radiation therapy based on deep learning. *Med. Phys.* **2023**, *50*, 284–296. [CrossRef]
42. Shanbhag, N.M.; Bin Sumaida, A.; Binz, T.; Hasnain, S.M.; El-Koha, O.; Al Kaabi, K.; Saleh, M.; Al Qawasmeh, K.; Balaraj, K. Integrating Artificial Intelligence into Radiation Oncology: Can Humans Spot AI? *Cureus* **2023**, *15*, e50486. [CrossRef] [PubMed]
43. Lustberg, T.; Van Soest, J.; Gooding, M.; Peressutti, D.; Aljabar, P.; Van Der Stoep, J.; Van Elmpt, W.; Dekker, A. Clinical evaluation of atlas and deep learning based automatic contouring for lung cancer. *Radiother. Oncol.* **2017**, *126*, 312–317. [CrossRef] [PubMed]
44. Cao, H.; Liu, H.; Song, E.; Hung, C.-C.; Ma, G.; Xu, X.; Jin, R.; Lu, J. Dual-branch residual network for lung nodule segmentation. *Appl. Soft Comput.* **2019**, *86*, 105934. [CrossRef]
45. Ning, Y.; Teixayavong, S.; Shang, Y.; Savulescu, J.; Nagaraj, V.; Miao, D.; Mertens, M.; Ting, D.S.W.; Ong, J.C.L.; Liu, M.; et al. Generative artificial intelligence and ethical considerations in health care: A scoping review and ethics checklist. *Lancet Digit. Health* **2024**, *6*, e848–e856. [CrossRef]
46. Automatic Contouring for Radiation Therapy. Available online: https://limbus.ai/ (accessed on 17 April 2024).
47. Hoque, S.M.H.; Pirrone, G.; Matrone, F.; Donofrio, A.; Fanetti, G.; Caroli, A.; Rista, R.S.; Bortolus, R.; Avanzo, M.; Drigo, A.; et al. Clinical Use of a Commercial Artificial Intelligence-Based Software for Autocontouring in Radiation Therapy: Geometric Performance and Dosimetric Impact. *Cancers* **2023**, *15*, 5735. [CrossRef]
48. Wang, J.; Lu, J.; Qin, G.; Shen, L.; Sun, Y.; Ying, H.; Zhang, Z.; Hu, W. Technical Note: A deep learning-based autosegmentation of rectal tumors in MR images. *Med. Phys.* **2018**, *45*, 2560–2564. [CrossRef]

49. Ronneberger, O.; Fischer, P.; Brox, T. U-Net: Convolutional Networks for Biomedical Image Segmentation. In *Dans Lecture Notes in Computer Science*; Springer: Berlin/Heidelberg, Germany, 2015; pp. 234–241. [CrossRef]
50. Clark, K.; Vendt, B.; Smith, K.; Freymann, J.; Kirby, J.; Koppel, P.; Moore, S.; Phillips, S.; Maffitt, D.; Pringle, M.; et al. The Cancer Imaging Archive (TCIA): Maintaining and Operating a Public Information Repository. *J. Digit. Imaging* **2013**, *26*, 1045–1057. [CrossRef]
51. Zuley, M.L.; Jarosz, R.; Kirk, S.; Lee, Y.; Colen, R.; Garcia, K.; Delbeke, D.; Pham, M.; Nagy, P.; Sevinc, G.; et al. The Cancer Genome Atlas Head-Neck Squamous Cell Carcinoma Collection (TCGA-HNSC) (Version 6) [Data set]. In *The Cancer Imaging Archive*; University of Arkansas for Medical Sciences: Little Rock, AR, USA, 2023. [CrossRef]
52. Zuley, M.L.; Jarosz, R.; Drake, B.F.; Rancilio, D.; Klim, A.; Rieger-Christ, K.; Lemmerman, J. The Cancer Genome Atlas Prostate Adenocarcinoma Collection (TCGA-PRAD) (Version 4) [Data set]. In *The Cancer Imaging Archive*; University of Arkansas for Medical Sciences: Little Rock, AR, USA, 2016. [CrossRef]
53. Rezaei, M.; Mohammadbeigi, A.; Khoshgard, K.; Haghparast, A. CT images and radiotherapy treatment planning of patients with breast cancer: A dataset. *Data Brief* **2017**, *13*, 390–395. [CrossRef] [PubMed]
54. Brouwer, C.L.; Steenbakkers, R.J.; Van Den Heuvel, E.; Duppen, J.C.; Navran, A.; Bijl, H.P.; Chouvalova, O.; Burlage, F.R.; Meertens, H.; Langendijk, J.A.; et al. 3D Variation in delineation of head and neck organs at risk. *Radiat. Oncol.* **2012**, *7*, 32. [CrossRef]
55. Grégoire, V.; Ang, K.; Budach, W.; Grau, C.; Hamoir, M.; Langendijk, J.A.; Lee, A.; Le, Q.-T.; Maingon, P.; Nutting, C.; et al. Delineation of the neck node levels for head and neck tumors: A 2013 update. DAHANCA, EORTC, HKNPCSG, NCIC CTG, NCRI, RTOG, TROG consensus guidelines. *Radiother. Oncol.* **2013**, *110*, 172–181. [CrossRef]
56. Sun, Y.; Yu, X.-L.; Luo, W.; Lee, A.W.M.; Wee, J.T.S.; Lee, N.; Zhou, G.-Q.; Tang, L.-L.; Tao, C.-J.; Guo, R.; et al. Recommendation for a contouring method and atlas of organs at risk in nasopharyngeal carcinoma patients receiving intensity-modulated radiotherapy. *Radiother. Oncol.* **2014**, *110*, 390–397. [CrossRef]
57. Gay, H.A.; Barthold, H.J.; O'Meara, E.; Bosch, W.R.; Naqa, I.E.; Al-Lozi, R.; Rosenthal, S.A.; Lawton, C.; Lee, W.R.; Sandler, H.; et al. Pelvic Normal Tissue Contouring Guidelines for Radiation Therapy: A Radiation Therapy Oncology Group Consensus Panel Atlas. *Int. J. Radiat. Oncol. Biol. Phys.* **2012**, *83*, e353–e362. [CrossRef] [PubMed]
58. Brouwer, C.L.; Steenbakkers, R.J.H.M.; Bourhis, J.; Budach, W.; Grau, C.; Grégoire, V.; Van Herk, M.; Lee, A.; Maingon, P.; Nutting, C.; et al. CT-based delineation of organs at risk in the head and neck region: DAHANCA, EORTC, GORTEC, HKNPCSG, NCIC CTG, NCRI, NRG Oncology and TROG consensus guidelines. *Radiother. Oncol.* **2015**, *117*, 83–90. [CrossRef]
59. Abadi, M.; Agarwal, A.; Barham, P.; Brevdo, E.; Chen, Z.; Citro, C.; Corrado, G.S.; Davis, A.; Dean, J.; Devin, M.; et al. TensorFlow: Large-Scale Machine Learning on Heterogeneous Distributed Systems. *arXiv* **2016**, arXiv:1603.04467. [CrossRef]
60. Zabel, W.J.; Conway, J.L.; Gladwish, A.; Skliarenko, J.; Didiodato, G.; Goorts-Matthews, L.; Michalak, A.; Reistetter, S.; King, J.; Nakonechny, K.; et al. Clinical Evaluation of Deep Learning and Atlas-Based Auto-Contouring of Bladder and Rectum for Prostate Radiation Therapy. *Pract. Radiat. Oncol.* **2021**, *11*, e80–e89. [CrossRef] [PubMed]
61. Gambacorta, M.A.; Chiloiro, G.; Valentini, V. Should We Tailor the Delineation of Pelvic Structures According to Tumor Presentation? In *Dans Springer eBooks*; Springer: Berlin/Heidelberg, Germany, 2018; pp. 165–179. [CrossRef]
62. Van Dijk, L.V.; Van Den Bosch, L.; Aljabar, P.; Peressutti, D.; Both, S.; Steenbakkers, R.J.; Langendijk, J.A.; Gooding, M.J.; Brouwer, C.L. Improving automatic delineation for head and neck organs at risk by Deep Learning Contouring. *Radiother. Oncol.* **2019**, *142*, 115–123. [CrossRef] [PubMed]
63. Oktay, O.; Nanavati, J.; Schwaighofer, A.; Carter, D.; Bristow, M.; Tanno, R.; Jena, R.; Barnett, G.; Noble, D.; Rimmer, Y.; et al. Evaluation of Deep Learning to Augment Image-Guided Radiotherapy for Head and Neck and Prostate Cancers. *JAMA Netw. Open* **2020**, *3*, e2027426. [CrossRef]
64. Kim, Y.W.; Biggs, S.; Mackonis, E.C. Investigation on performance of multiple AI-based auto-contouring systems in organs at risks (OARs) delineation. *Phys. Eng. Sci. Med.* **2024**, *47*, 1123–1140. [CrossRef]
65. Wong, W.K.; Leung, L.H.; Kwong, D.L. Evaluation and optimization of the parameters used in multiple-atlas-based segmentation of prostate cancers in radiation therapy. *Br. J. Radiol.* **2016**, *89*, 20140732. [CrossRef]
66. Doolan, P.J.; Charalambous, S.; Roussakis, Y.; Leczynski, A.; Peratikou, M.; Benjamin, M.; Ferentinos, K.; Strouthos, I.; Zamboglou, C.; Karagiannis, E. A clinical evaluation of the performance of five commercial artificial intelligence contouring systems for radiotherapy. *Front. Oncol.* **2023**, *13*, 1213068. [CrossRef]
67. Fan, M.; Wang, T.; Lei, Y.; Patel, P.R.; Dresser, S.; Ghavidel, B.B.; Qiu, R.L.J.; Zhou, J.; Luca, K.; Kayode, O.; et al. Evaluation and failure analysis of four commercial deep learning-based autosegmentation software for abdominal organs at risk. *J. Appl. Clin. Med. Phys.* **2025**, *26*, e70010. [CrossRef] [PubMed]

Current Oncology MDPI

Article

Focal Therapy for Localized Prostate Cancer: A Case Series with Cost Analysis

Maxwell Sandberg [1,2,*], David Thole [1], Jackson Nowatzke [1], Gavin Underwood [1], Emily Ye [1], Soroush Rais-Bahrami [1,2], Ronald Davis [1,2] and Alejandro Rodriguez [1,2]

1 Department of Urology, Wake Forest University School of Medicine, Winston Salem, NC 27101, USA; david.thole@wfusm.edu (D.T.); jackson.nowatzke@wfusm.edu (J.N.); gavin.underwood@wfusm.edu (G.U.); emily.ye@wfusm.edu (E.Y.); soroush.raisbahrami@advocatehealth.org (S.R.-B.); ronald.l.davis@advocatehealth.edu (R.D.); alejandro.rodriguez@advocatehealth.org (A.R.)

2 Comprehensive Cancer Center, Atrium Health Wake Forest Baptist Medical Center, Winston Salem, NC 27101, USA

* Correspondence: maxwell.sandberg@advocatehealth.org; Tel.: +1-248-904-5200

Simple Summary: Prostate cancer treatment has shifted dramatically over the last decade. In this manuscript, a case series of three different focal therapy modalities (high-intensity focused ultrasound, cryoablation, and irreversible electroporation of the prostate) to treat prostate cancer is reported. The analysis compares functional and oncologic controls. Focal therapy provides adequate functional outcomes with oncologic control like established whole-gland therapies. Additionally, the cost by treatment modality is compared, often disregarded when considering focal therapy. Lastly, a brief narrative review of the literature was conducted to contextualize our findings.

Abstract: Focal therapy for prostate cancer (PCa) provides approaches to treat PCa patients in a less invasive manner than traditional whole-gland surgical or radiation modalities. This manuscript provides a case series of high-intensity focused ultrasound (HIFU), cryoablation, and irreversible electroporation (IRE) for PCa at a single institution and cost analysis with a review of the literature. All patients who underwent HIFU, cryoablation, or IRE for localized PCa were retrospectively reviewed, excluding patients who received whole-gland therapy. Functional outcomes were erectile dysfunction and lower urinary tract symptoms. Cost data were collected. A total of 45 patients were included in the study with focal therapy ranging from 2023 to 2025 (4 HIFU, 20 cryoablation, 21 IRE). A total of 30 patients had focally treated lesions, and 15 patients had hemi-gland treatment. The mean preoperative PSA was 7.7 ng/mL. On the paired sample t-test, there was no significant difference between pre-focal and post-focal therapy PSA. Three patients experienced biochemical recurrence requiring prostate biopsy after focal treatment. Mean cost was USD 3804.50 and not significantly different by focal treatment. No metastatic events occurred nor deaths at a median follow-up of 6 months. Patients in this series had largely unaltered functional outcomes. Cost analysis in contemporary publications is lacking. Although follow-up was short, cancer control was adequate.

Keywords: focal; prostate cancer; HIFU; IRE; cryoablation

1. Introduction

The annual rate of incidence of prostate cancer (PCa) in the United States of America (USA) was over 299,000 in the year 2024 [1]. PCa treatments have been revolutionized over the last decade, with improved survival rates. In 2024, the five-year cancer-specific survival (CSS) was estimated to be 97% in the USA alone [1]. Traditional treatments for PCa have been radical prostatectomy (RP) and radiation to the prostate, each of which is a whole-gland therapy with curative intent, still widely employed in practice today. The literature varies, but approximately 40–60% of men opt for RP as the primary means to treat their PCa [2–4]. The average number of RP performed in the USA has remained relatively steady but difficult to estimate, at around 138,000 RP performed each year [5]. However, only a minority of urologists are high-volume surgeons performing the majority of RP [6]. The second most common treatment selection is radiation therapy, either external beam radiation or brachytherapy approaches directed by radiation oncologists, with approximately 37% of men with PCa receiving primary radiation therapy each year for their disease [4]. Both RP and radiation therapy carry significant side effects to patients. These are most often urinary incontinence and erectile dysfunction (ED). ED and urinary incontinence can impact upwards of 30% and upwards of 70–80% of patients after RP, respectively [7]. Further, evidence has pointed to around 30% of patients experiencing urinary incontinence and 30–50% of patients experiencing ED after radiation therapy [8]. Only ~5–10% of PCa patients elect active surveillance in the USA, although the number is significantly higher for low-risk disease, with some estimating 60% [9,10]. This is particularly relevant as 10–30% of patients with localized PCa report regret in the way they managed their PCa [11,12]. There are multiple reasons for this but given there is still a 2.6% risk of dying of PCa, many men want to take a more active role in treating their disease but may not be aware of the side effects with the standard whole-gland treatment options [13]. Additionally, the increased use of prostate indication magnetic resonance imaging (MRI) and MRI-guided biopsy through software fusion technologies has augmented the reliability of grade and stage-defining diagnostic biopsy samples, with more confident decision making when suitable for surveillance versus definitive therapy of varying levels of aggressiveness [14–16].

Focal therapy with various ablative energy sources has created a revolutionary approach to managing PCa in a less invasive way. Subtotal gland treatments can use a variety of different energy modalities, all with the fundamental goals of treating index lesions of known, localized PCa while sparing unaffected tissue regions in the gland [17]. Often, this includes but is not limited to high-intensity focused ultrasound (HIFU), cryotherapy, and irreversible electroporation (IRE) of the prostate which have long been used and vetted for whole-gland prostate ablative approaches [18]. There is a paucity of research comparing these different modalities, and no randomized clinical trial exists comparing them head-to-head with standard-of-care, whole-gland curative treatment options (RP or radiation therapy) [19]. Current case series seem to show promising results for HIFU, cryoablation, and IRE with respect to functional outcome preservation in focal treatments [19–21]. Cancer control evidence is not as strong for focal treatments, but case series in the literature seem to show no difference in overall survival (OS) and metastasis-free survival (MFS) compared to RP and radiation [19]. Nevertheless, additional patient data is required, and cost is not factored into many of the contemporary publications of these treatment modalities. The purpose of this paper is to report a case series of focal/hemi-gland HIFU, cryoablation, and IRE with respect to functional outcomes and cost at a single institution and provide a brief narrative review of the literature surrounding these treatment modalities. Secondarily, the purpose was to report short-term oncologic outcomes.

2. Materials and Methods

This was a retrospective study from 2023 to 2025 performed at a single institution of all patients who underwent either HIFU, cryoablation, and/or IRE for localized PCa. All patients who received whole-gland therapy were excluded, such that only focal and/or hemi-gland therapy was included in the analysis. The study was approved under the Wake Forest Baptist Institutional Review Board (IRB00132775). Demographic information was collected on all eligible participants including age, race, comorbidities, and Charlson Comorbidity Index (CCI) at the time of focal therapy administration. Functional status at baseline was tracked for both ED and lower urinary tract symptoms (LUTS). This was achieved in the form of both qualitative documentation of ED and LUTS preoperatively as well as preoperative International Index of Erectile Function (IIEF) scores and International Prostatic Symptom Scores (IPSS). Additionally, complications were recorded after focal therapy and graded using the Clavien-Dindo classification system [22]. Preoperative oncologic data were also collected which included prior prostate biopsy data with grade group (GG) prior to therapy, prostate-specific antigen (PSA) value prior to focal treatment, prostate size on MRI, and prior history of focal treatment and/or other treatment for PCa. Patients were also categorized based on PCa risk category using the American Urologic Association Classification System [23]. Patient selection for focal therapy was at surgeon discretion and not standardized in the study. However, it was most often based on GG and PCa risk stratification, with a specific focus on GG 1–2 and risk category $\leq$ favorable intermediate risk. All patients were required to have a pre-focal therapy MRI completed, most often within 3 months or less of focal therapy administration, all of which were multiparametric MRIs. There were no absolute exclusions by tumor location, but multiple positive locales on preoperative prostate biopsy were typically justified by a surgeon for hemi-gland over focal gland treatment. There were no criteria to choose one energy modality over another (i.e., cryoablation versus IRE, etc.). However, HIFU was only recently introduced to this institution in 2024, which accounts for its making up the smallest proportion of patients in the study. HIFU was performed using Sonablate® (Charlotte, NC, USA), IRE was performed using NanoKnife systems, and cryoablation was performed through Endocare™ (CryoCare CS®, Winston Salem, NC, USA) and Galil (Boston Scientific, Winston Salem, NC, USA) probes.

Postoperative oncologic data recorded included operative time, most recent follow-up PSA, need for additional prostate biopsy and biopsy data, development of metastasis, most recent follow-up, and OS. All patients were seen in the clinic postoperatively 4–6 weeks after focal therapy administration with a PSA lab draw. Then, a PSA was followed at 3, 6, and 12 months post-procedure. An MRI was performed one year post-therapy. A post-treatment confirmatory biopsy was performed based upon the PSA and MRI results, specifically using MRI targeting of any sites of suspicion and the site of post-ablative tissue involution changes. PSA was then checked every 6 months up to 5 years post-focal therapy. The postoperative PSA median follow-up interval was six months. Cost data was obtained from medical record logs of each case and comprised healthcare system costs, not costs to the patient. This included operating room disposable costs such as supplies, machinery (which was rented now owned), and the like. Operating room block times and anesthesia costs were not included. Not every case had available cost data, so only cases with cost information (IRE and cryoablation) were included in the analysis on cost. Additionally, not every patient had a complete set of data available in the electronic medical record. Independent sample t-test was utilized to compare the mean cost between IRE and cryoablation. Analysis of variance was used to compare operative time by treatment modality. Paired sample t-test was used to compare pre-focal to post-focal therapy PSA values both in the overall cohort and for each individual treatment type. All statistical analysis was performed using SPSS Statistics Version 28 (Armonk, NY, USA).

In addition to reporting a case series, this study performed a brief review of the literature and summarized these findings in the discussion of the paper. Further, the data from this case series were compared in descriptive format to some current publications.

3. Results

A total of 45 patients were included in the analysis (4 HIFU, 20 cryoablation, and 21 IRE; Table 1). Of these, 30 patients had focally treated lesions, and 15 patients had hemi-gland treatment. Median follow-up was 6 months in the study. The mean age at the time of focal therapy was 70.1 years old. There were 34 (76%) Caucasian patients, 8 (18%) patients who were black, and 3 (7%) patients whose race was listed as "other." Mean CCI was 5.7 at the time of focal therapy. A total of 13 (29%) patients received prior treatment for their PCa. Of these, two had brachytherapy, four had radiation therapy, six had prior cryoablation, and one had prior IRE. Focal therapy is not infrequently administered in the salvage setting after prior treatment for PCa rather than as a primary treatment, with promising outcomes for use in this setting; thus, it was deemed justified to include these patients in the study [24–26]. Further, the goal of this paper was to report a case series of HIFU, cryoablation, and IRE which provided additional justification for their inclusion. There were 27 (60%) patients with ED preoperatively and 16 (36%) patients noted to have ED postoperatively. The mean preoperative IIEF score was 14.7, and the mean postoperative IIEF score was 7. Two patients did not have ED pre-focal therapy and were found to have developed ED post-focal therapy in the study (1 IRE and 1 cryoablation). There were 23 (51%) patients noted to have LUTS preoperatively and 20 (44%) patients with LUTS postoperatively. The mean preoperative IPSS was 7.9, and the mean postoperative IPSS was 6. Five patients with no LUTS pre-focal therapy developed LUTS post-focal therapy (two IRE and three cryoablation). The mean prostate size at the time of treatment was 46.1 cc. Figure 1 displays an algorithm for urologists to use when considering focal therapy for a patient with PCa.

Table 1. Focal therapy series data. The following table shows different patient and oncologic variables in the left-most column. Each focal modality is shown with corresponding values for each variable. Continuous variables are means with standard deviations in parentheses. Categorical variables are total numbers with percentage of the cohort in parentheses. Total represents the entire focal therapy cohort.

Variable	HIFU	IRE	Cryoablation	Total
N	4	21	20	45
Age	66.5 (13.3)	70.5 (7.4)	70.6 (7.4)	70.1 (8.2)
Caucasian Black Other	3 (75) 1 (25) 0	16 (76) 5 (24) 0	15 (75) 2 (10) 3 (15)	34 (76) 8 (18) 3 (7)
Charlson Comorbidity	4 (5.0)	5.7(1.7)	5.9 (2.0)	5.7 (1.9)
IIEF preoperative	19.5 (0.7)	13.6 (7.3)	14.7 (8.3)	14.7 (7.4)
ED preoperative	1 (25)	12 (57)	14 (70)	27 (60)
IPSS preoperative	7.3 (4.6)	8.1 (3.5)	8.0 (7.4)	7.9 (5.2)
LUTS preoperative	2 (50)	11 (52)	10 (50)	23 (51)

Table 1. *Cont.*

Variable	HIFU	IRE	Cryoablation	Total
Focal	1 (25)	17 (81)	12 (60)	30 (67)
Hemi	3 (75)	4 (19)	8 (40)	15 (33)
Prior treatment				
Brachytherapy	0 (0)	0 (0)	2 (10)	2 (15)
Radiation	0 (0)	1 (5)	3 (15)	4 (31)
Cryoablation	0 (0)	2 (10)	4 (20)	6 (46)
IRE	0 (0)	0 (0)	1 (5)	1 (8)
Preoperative PSA (ng/mL)	7.2 (2.2)	7.0 (3.0)	8.5 (3.8)	7.7 (3.3)
GG preoperative				
1	0 (0)	2 (10)	3 (15)	5 (11)
2	3 (75)	13 (62)	14 (70)	30 (67)
3	1 (25)	5 (24)	3 (15)	9 (20)
4	0 (0)	1 (5)	0 (0)	1 (2)
Prostate size (cc)	52.8 (17.3)	51.3 (25.4)	39.5 (17.0)	46.1 (21.7)
Very low risk	0	2	2	4 (9)
Favorable intermediate risk	5	13	17	35 (78)
Unfavorable intermediate risk	1	5	3	9 (20)
High risk	0	1	0	1 (2)
Operative time (minutes)	114.3 (20.6)	43.1 (6.1)	65.2 (14.0)	59.2 (23.3)
Complication	1 (25)	7 (33)	8 (40)	16 (36)
Clavien				
I	0 (0)	4 (19)	5 (25)	
II	2 (50)	3 (14)	1 (5)	9 (20)
IIIa	0 (0)	0 (0)	2 (10)	6 (13)
IIIb	0 (0)	0 (0)	0 (0)	2 (4)
IV	0 (0)	0 (0)	0 (0)	
V	0 (0)	0 (0)	0 (0)	
Most recent PSA (ng/mL)	4.5 (2.4)	3.5 (2.4)	2.5 (2.2)	3.1 (2.3)
Biopsy postoperative	0 (0)	0 (0)	3 (15)	3 (7)
Positive biopsy postoperative	0 (0)	0 (0)	3 (15)	3 (7)
GG postoperative	-	-	3 (100)	3 (100)
IIEF postoperative	-	14 (67)	7	10.5 (5)
ED postoperative	0 (0)	4 (19)	12 (60)	16 (36)
IPSS postoperative	5	0	6.3 (6.8)	6 (5.6)
LUTS postoperative	0 (0)	7 (33)	13 (65)	20 (44)
Cost (USD)	-	3762.3 (2552.3)	4648.3	3804.5 (2495.2)
Metastasis	0	0	0	-
Dead	0	0	0	-
Follow-up (months)	4 (3–8)	4 (4–7)	12 (2.5–17)	6 (3–12)

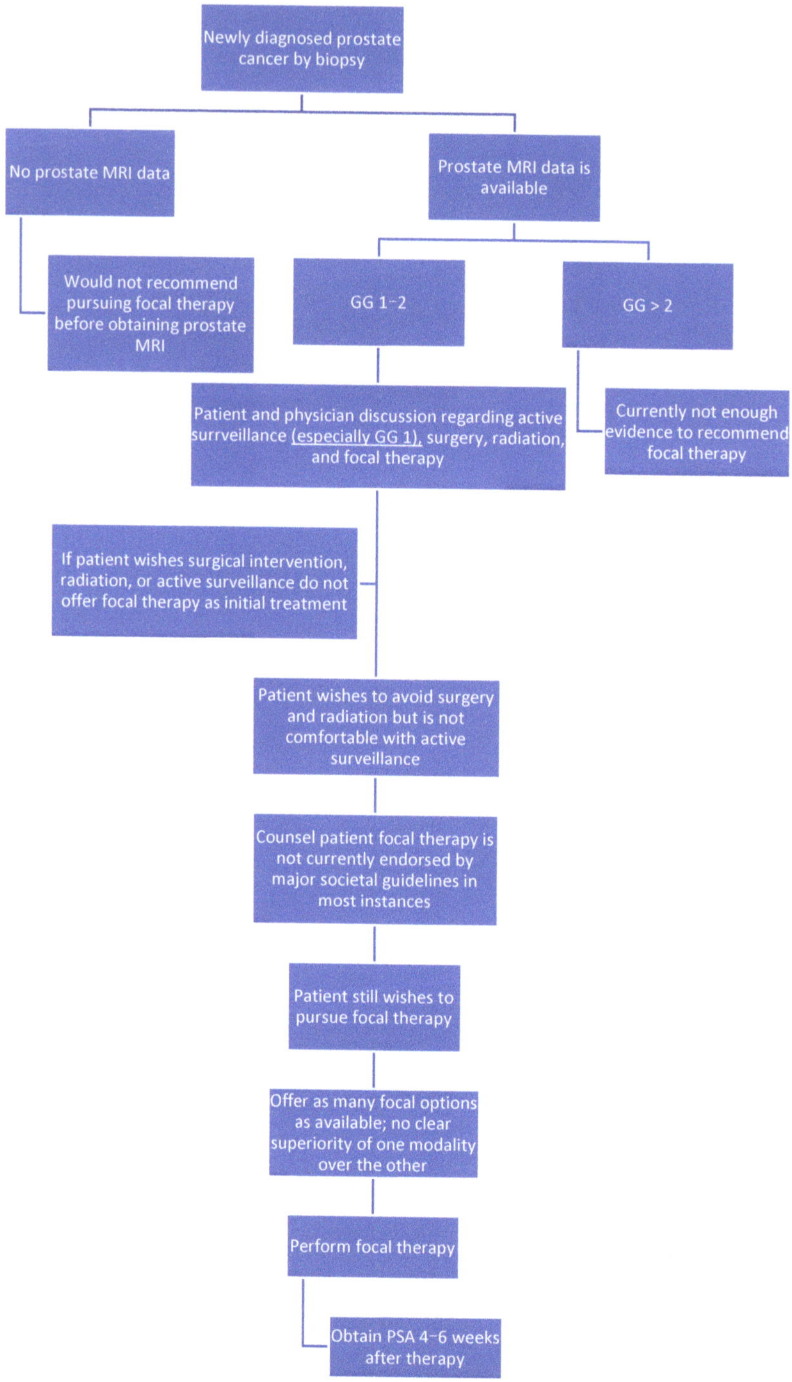

Figure 1. Focal therapy algorithm. The following image displays an algorithm generated by the authors of this manuscript to guide urologists considering focal therapy for a patient with prostate cancer. It is not meant to represent level I evidence nor expert-agreed fact. This algorithm also does not address salvage focal therapy in the setting of previously treated prostate cancer.

Mean preoperative PSA was 7.7 ng/mL. There were 5 (11%) patients with GG 1 PCa preoperatively, 30 (67%) patients with GG2 PCa, 9 (20%) patients with GG3 PCa, and 1 (2%) patient with GG4 PCa. There were 4 (9%) patients with very low risk PCa, 35 (78%) patients with favorable intermediate risk PCa, 9 (20%) patients with unfavorable intermediate risk PCa, and 1 (2%) patient with high risk PCa preoperatively in the cohort. The mean operative time was 59.2 min overall, with a significant difference by focal modality with HIFU at 114.3 min, cryoablation at 65.2 min, and IRE at 43.1 min ($p < 0.05$). Overall, there were 16 (36%) complications reported postoperatively. Of these, only two were > Clavien-Dindo II, and both were IIIa. The most recent mean PSA on follow-up was 3.1 ng/mL. On the paired sample t-test, there was no significant difference between pre-focal and post-focal therapy PSA ($p > 0.05$; Table 2). In individual focal therapy analysis, both IRE and cryoablation had a significantly lower PSA post-focal therapy compared to pre-focal therapy ($p < 0.05$), but HIFU did not ($p > 0.05$). There were three patients who underwent postoperative biopsy after focal therapy during the study window, all of whom were cryoablation patients, and all of whom were positive for PCa. All biopsies (100%) were GG2 disease. No patients died during the study window nor did anybody develop metastasis.

Table 2. Paired samples t-test for PSA. The following table compares pre-focal therapy PSA to post-focal therapy PSA values. Each individual treatment modality is shown along with the total cohort. *p*-values are provided for reference.

Therapy	PSA Preoperative (ng/mL)	PSA Postoperative (ng/mL)	*p*-Value
HIFU	6.4 (1.9)	4.5 (2.4)	0.082
IRE	7.1 (3.3)	3.5 (2.4)	0.001
Cryoablation	8.0 (3.8)	2.5 (2.2)	<0.001
Total	7.5 (3.4)	3.1 (2.3)	0.854

Cost data was only available for IRE and cryoablation patients. Mean cost of IRE was USD 3762.30 and mean cost of cryoablation was USD 4648.30 ($p > 0.05$).

4. Discussion

Currently, focal therapy is not endorsed by the American Urologic Association and National Comprehensive Cancer Network (NCCN) guidelines to treat PCa for any risk level, aside from select instances of radio-recurrent PCa [23,27,28]. If a patient fails radiation therapy for PCa and has a recurrence, whole-gland cryoablation and HIFU are considered for salvage treatment in the NCCN guidelines [27,28]. The European Association of Urology guidelines note that HIFU and cryoablation may be considered for select patients as part of a clinical trial or prospective cohort study [29,30]. Recently, the FocAL therapy CONsensus (FALCON) project released some recommendations to refine partial gland ablation for localized prostate cancer [31,32]. Although no consensus or significant societal endorsement exists for focal therapy in PCa guidelines, many urologists employ these treatment modalities in select cases, largely with the driver of patient desire and the advances in pretreatment imaging defining the isolated localization of clinically significant PCa foci [33,34].

There is a paucity of data on the exact percentage of patients opting for focal therapy to treat their PCa, with some critics noting its use in improperly selected patients. In Germany, Flegar et al. analyzed the German Billing Database for focal therapy over the course of 2006–2019 for hyperthermia ablation, cryoablation, vascular-targeted photodynamic therapy, transurethral ultrasound ablation, and various other modalities [35]. They found nearly 24,000 focal therapy cases for PCa performed in this time frame, with an initial increase and then a plateau in use around the year 2015. However, for patients >70 years old undergoing focal treatment for PCa, they noted a significant increase over time in its use [35]. Interestingly, the mean age in this series was >70 years old. Multiple critics of focal therapy argue that it is too often employed to treat disease in the wrong patients or undertreats clinically significant PCa [36,37]. Tay et al. performed a systematic analysis of HIFU, cryoablation, and IRE [38]. They noted an increasing trend of these treatments being used for GG2-5 disease and a downtrend in their use for GG1 PCa in their study. At this institution, there has been an uptick in HIFU, which was only added as an option for patients under care early in 2024, as well as increased utilization of IRE. Further, only 11% of this case series received treatment for primary pattern GG1 disease. The data highlights the need for large population-based studies to identify how frequently focal therapy is being employed and in which patients urologists are opting to use it on.

Functional outcomes were adequate, like much of the current literature. Proponents of treatments like HIFU, cryoablation, and IRE argue improved ED and lesser degrees of LUTS relative to radical surgery or radiation in PCa [37]. Just two patients who did not have ED preoperatively were found to have developed it after therapy. Tay et al. performed a systematic review of 49 HIFU, cryotherapy, and IRE studies, of which 35 reported sexual function data [38]. The overwhelming majority of studies reported a low to moderate impact of all three treatments on sexual function, with only two studies reporting severe sexual side effects. Additionally, no significant differences were identified between each of the three treatments. While this study did not directly compare each focal modality in the case series, similar proportions of patients with ED pre- and post-focal therapy by treatment modality were identified. Another review by Hopstaken et al. included 27 HIFU studies, 11 on cryoablation, and 9 on IRE [39]. These authors broke HIFU down to a prior history of transurethral resection of the prostate (TURP) versus no prior TURP, as some perform TURP initially to reduce the risk of urinary retention. For HIFU with TURP, sexual function was mixed, with some authors noting a moderate increase in ED after HIFU, while others showed a return to baseline one year postoperatively [40–42]. For patients who had HIFU and no prior TURP history, a median decrease in erectile function of 12% was noted after HIFU, and there was a median increase in the use of phosphodiesterase five inhibitors (17%) after treatment [39]. No patients in this HIFU series had a TURP prior. For IRE, six of the nine studies in Hopstaken's review noted ED after therapy, and 50% of these reported severe dysfunction [39]. One important analysis by Mendez et al. compared focal to whole-gland cryoablation, noting significantly improved sexual function in focally treated patients, with nearly 50% reporting early return to sexual activity [43]. Tan et al. published on 28 patients who underwent focal cryoablation, concluding there was a transient decline in sexual function postoperatively, but this recovered within three months [44]. Rastinehad et al. found that out of 282 focal cryoablation patients, 74% of patients potent prior to therapy maintained erections necessary for sexual intercourse after cryoablation [45]. In this series, 67% of patients received focal gland therapy compared to 33% hemi-gland.

Urinary outcomes for focal HIFU, cryoablation, and IRE vary across the literature, but appear comparable to those of RP or radiation. In this study's cohort, nearly identical rates of LUTS before and after focal therapy were seen. Additionally, only two patients who did not report LUTS before focal therapy were found to have developed LUTS postoperatively. In ten studies of TURP followed by HIFU, 95% of patients were pad-free after HIFU [39]. For HIFU without TURP, nearly 96% of patients in six different studies were pad-free after treatment [39]. IRE had even better outcomes in the analysis by Hopstaken et al., with a 100% pad-free rate. Other contemporary series on IRE report continence rates also approaching 100%, although one small series of elderly patients noted pads to be required in 18% of patients more than six months postoperatively [46]. Looking at cryoablation, Hopstaken et al.'s meta-analysis had five focal studies reporting urinary continence outcomes, of which four noted 100% pad-free continence after therapy [39]. Mendez et al. compared focal to whole-gland cryoablation, finding improved urinary continence rates in the focal grouping [43]. Rastinehead et al. recently presented a cohort of 282 patients who underwent focal cryoablation for PCa, with a 98% pad-free rate at 12 months postoperatively [45]. In summary, it appears IRE offers the highest rates of continence postoperatively of the three modalities, but all provide adequate outcomes in this domain. IRE patients in this series had outcomes in line with this, but given the small cohort and follow-up, no definitive comments on the superiority of one focal therapy over another using these data can be made.

Oncologic outcomes for HIFU, cryotherapy, and IRE are difficult to assess due to significant heterogeneity in the current study design and patient selection. Nevertheless, the current landscape seems to indicate that outcomes are adequate. In Tay et al.'s systematic analysis of HIFU, cryoablation, and IRE, 22 different studies reported survival outcomes, with 98% OS noted [38]. CSS was 99.3%. MFS was 98.5%, and no difference in OS, CSS, or MFS was observed by focal modality [38]. Additionally, biochemical recurrence was noted to be approximately 9% per year. Ślusarczyk et al. performed a meta-analysis of prospective focal therapy studies, which included 50 studies, of which 18 were HIFU, 11 cryoablation, and 7 IRE [47]. The 12-month biopsy-proven recurrence-free survival was 81% and was not different by focal therapy type. MFS differed based on median follow-up in the study but ranged from 93 to 100%. Most research did not directly compare oncologic outcomes by focal therapy type, but Stabile et al. compared HIFU to cryoablation and did not identify oncologic superiority of one modality over the other [48]. No deaths occurred in this analysis's study window nor metastatic events. The short follow-up time and heterogeneous cohort make oncologic analysis complicated. The overall body of literature, however, appears promising.

Adverse events in Ślusarczyk et al.'s study found complications $\geq$ Clavien III in approximately 3% of instances, with no difference by focal modality [47]. Hopstaken et al. reported a median $\geq$ Clavien III complication rate of 1.9% in HIFU with TURP, 2% in HIFU without TURP, cryoablation ranged with most studies noting 0–1.6%, and nearly 0% for IRE [39]. In this study, a complication rate of 35% was noted, but only 4% of complications were $\geq$Clavien III, all of which were IIIa. Given that RP has a complication rate $\geq$ Clavien III around 9%, focal therapy appears to be a safe alternative for clinicians to employ [49].

One of the main issues with focal ablative therapy is the lack of level one evidence to allow for adoption in the large panel-derived guideline bodies that define its role in the treatment of PCa. No clinical trial has ever been published directly comparing focal therapy to RP or whole-gland radiation therapy. The only randomized clinical trial to compare focal therapy to standard-of-care treatments in the space of PCa evaluated 206 men who received vascular targeted photodynamic therapy of the prostate to 207 men on active surveillance [50]. There was a significantly lower rate of disease progression in the phototherapy group relative to active surveillance and at a four-year lower rate of requiring radical therapy [50,51]. Clinical trial design is difficult. The correct target population to include in the ideal clinical trial remains elusive. Additionally, as noted by others, even the best focal therapy studies have only modest population sizes [52]. Further, treating localized tumor lesions does not necessarily lead to meaningful survival outcomes [52]. Questions also remain regarding future urologists using focal therapy in their practices, as little data exists on how often urologic residents receive exposure and if they are even trained in it at all.

A unique aspect of this case series is the inclusion of cost data. Most of the cost information came from IRE, which was found not to significantly differ from cryoablation. Consideration should be given to the difference in operative time, appreciated though, as IRE had the shortest operative time. Reddy et al. utilized a Markov Model to model stable disease, local recurrence, metastatic disease, and death from PCa [53]. Focal therapy was defined as either cryoablation or HIFU, and radical therapy was RP or radiation. Interestingly, focal therapy had lower overall costs and higher quality-adjusted life year gains compared to RP or radiation [53]. Silva and Lima calculated that it costs around USD 1100 to treat a man with PCa using HIFU [54]. There is surprisingly little published data comparing focal therapy modalities by cost to one another. Given that there does not appear to be a meaningful difference by focal therapy regarding functional outcomes nor cancer control, cost should be a high priority when considering treating a patient with either HIFU, cryoablation, or IRE.

Multiple limitations exist in this series worth acknowledging. First, while the majority of the literature is mainly small cohorts of focal therapy patients, this study also has relatively small numbers of patients who received HIFU, cryoablation, and IRE. Moreover, the short interval of follow-up significantly limits the study's ability to analyze functional and oncologic outcomes. The limited follow-up particularly limits oncologic data, as it is unexpected that relevant outcomes like recurrence or metastasis would frequently happen in the 6-month median follow-up time. Focal therapy is relatively new and has been slow to be adopted in mainstream practice, and short follow-up times are relatively ubiquitous in the literature, with many studies reporting median follow-ups of less than two years [24]. An updated series with lengthier follow-ups would be useful in the future to report on. A complete set of data, both pre- and post-focal therapy on each patient (i.e., IIEF scores, IPSS, etc.) for the entire series, was not available, given the retrospective nature of the data collection. Additionally, there are other ablative modalities used for focal therapy that are not included in the current analysis and literature review since they are not currently offered in this institution's practice including laser ablation, focal brachytherapy, focal stereotactic body radiation therapy, and partial prostatectomy. The cost information included is a strength of this series, but no cost data were available for HIFU patients, and minimal data were available on cryoablation. Further, costs were mainly representative of operating room disposables and machinery rentals, so it is likely the analysis underestimates the true total cost of focal therapy. Moreover, given that wage levels, material prices, and other factors vary across countries and regions, the conclusions of this study only represent the results from a single institution where the study was conducted. Therefore, the cost significance of this study is limited. Still, given the paucity of cost analysis in the focal therapy literature, there is still value in this data which can guide more robust studies in the future.

5. Conclusions

In this case series, outcomes of treating localized PCa patients with either HIFU, cryoablation, or IRE at a single institution were presented. Additionally, a comprehensive synopsis of the current literature surrounding these focal treatment options was conducted. Outcomes show focal therapy to be feasible, with excellent functional outcomes and adequate oncologic control. Moreover, cost was analyzed. The literature shows similar success with HIFU, cryoablation, and IRE. What is clear from this series and review is that more level one evidence evaluating focal therapy compared to the standard of care in PCa is required before fully implementing these therapies into guidelines. Nevertheless, they represent an exciting new avenue for future research, and focal therapy seems poised to change the landscape of PCa management moving forward.

Author Contributions: Conceptualization, M.S., D.T., J.N., G.U., E.Y., S.R.-B., R.D. and A.R.; methodology, M.S., S.R.-B., R.D. and A.R.; software, M.S., D.T., J.N., G.U. and E.Y.; validation, M.S., D.T., J.N., G.U., E.Y., S.R.-B., R.D. and A.R.; formal analysis, M.S.; investigation, M.S., D.T., J.N., G.U., E.Y., S.R.-B., R.D. and A.R.; resources, M.S., S.R.-B., R.D. and A.R.; data curation, M.S., D.T., J.N., G.U. and E.Y.; writing—original draft preparation, M.S., D.T., J.N., G.U., E.Y., S.R.-B., R.D. and A.R.; writing—review and editing, M.S., D.T., J.N., G.U., E.Y., S.R.-B., R.D. and A.R.; visualization, M.S.; supervision, R.D., S.R.-B. and A.R.; project administration, M.S. All authors have read and agreed to the published version of the manuscript.

Funding: This research received no external funding.

Institutional Review Board Statement: The study was conducted in accordance with the Declaration of Helsinki and approved by the Institutional Review Board (or Ethics Committee) of Wake Forest Baptist Institutional Review Board (IRB00132775, 12 December 2024).

Informed Consent Statement: Patient consent was waived due to the retrospective nature of this study.

Data Availability Statement: Data is not publicly available due to patient privacy, but will be made available in a de-identified format upon reasonable request to the corresponding author.

Conflicts of Interest: The authors declare no conflicts of interest.

Abbreviations

The following abbreviations are used in this manuscript:

PCa	Prostate cancer
USA	United States of America
RP	Radical prostatectomy
ED	Erectile dysfunction
MRI	Magnetic resonance imaging
HIFU	High-intensity focused ultrasound
IRE	Irreversible electroporation
OS	Overall survival
MFS	Metastasis-free survival
LUTS	Lower urinary tract symptoms
IIEF	International Index of Erectile Function
IPSS	International Prostatic Symptom Score
GG	Grade group
NCCN	National Comprehensive Cancer Network
FALCOS	FocAL therapy CONsensus
TURP	Transurethral resection of prostate
CSS	Cancer-specific survival

References

1. Siegel, R.L.; Giaquinto, A.N.; Jemal, A. Cancer statistics, 2024. *CA Cancer J. Clin.* **2024**, *74*, 12–49. [CrossRef]
2. Anandadas, C.N.; Clarke, N.W.; Davidson, S.E.; O'Reilly, P.H.; Logue, J.P.; Gilmore, L.; Swindell, R.; Brough, R.J.; Wemyss-Holden, G.D.; Lau, M.W.; et al. Early prostate cancer—Which treatment do men prefer and why? *BJU Int.* **2011**, *107*, 1762–1768. [CrossRef] [PubMed]
3. Kaps, B.; Leapman, M.; An, Y. Trends in prostatectomy utilization: Increasing upfront prostatectomy and postprostatectomy radiotherapy for high-risk prostate cancer. *Cancer Med.* **2020**, *9*, 8754–8764. [CrossRef]
4. Diven, M.A.; Tshering, L.; Ma, X.; Hu, J.C.; Barbieri, C.; McClure, T.; Nagar, H. Trends in Active Surveillance for Men with Intermediate-Risk Prostate Cancer. *JAMA Netw. Open* **2024**, *7*, e2429760. [CrossRef] [PubMed]
5. Oberlin, D.T.; Flum, A.S.; Lai, J.D.; Meeks, J.J. The effect of minimally invasive prostatectomy on practice patterns of American urologists. *Urol. Oncol.* **2016**, *34*, 255.e1–255.e5. [CrossRef] [PubMed]

6. Lee, D.; Tan, H.-J.; Fang, R.; Mbassa, R.; Matulewicz, R. Primary Question: How Has the Average Number of Radical Prostatectomies Performed by Urologists Changed Over Time? *AUA NEWS*, 25 October 2023. Available online: https://auanews.net/issues/articles/2023/october-extra-2023/primary-question-how-has-the-average-number-of-radical-prostatectomies-performed-by-urologists-changed-over-time (accessed on 19 June 2025).
7. Cornford, P.; van den Bergh, R.C.N.; Briers, E.; Van den Broeck, T.; Brunckhorst, O.; Darraugh, J.; Eberli, D.; De Meerleer, G.; De Santis, M.; Farolfi, A.; et al. EAU-EANM-ESTRO-ESUR-ISUP-SIOG Guidelines on Prostate Cancer-2024 Update. Part I: Screening, Diagnosis, and Local Treatment with Curative Intent. *Eur. Urol.* **2024**, *86*, 148–163. [CrossRef] [PubMed]
8. Muise, A.; Pan, M.M.; Rose, B.; Buckley, J.C. Functional outcomes after prostate cancer treatment: A comparison between single and multiple modalities. *Urol. Oncol.* **2023**, *41*, 104.e1–104.e9. [CrossRef] [PubMed]
9. Hayes, J.H.; Ollendorf, D.A.; Pearson, S.D.; Barry, M.J.; Kantoff, P.W.; Stewart, S.T.; Bhatnagar, V.; Sweeney, C.J.; Stahl, J.E.; McMahon, P.M. Active surveillance compared with initial treatment for men with low-risk prostate cancer: A decision analysis. *JAMA* **2010**, *304*, 2373–2380. [CrossRef] [PubMed]
10. Cooperberg, M.R.; Meeks, W.; Fang, R.; Gaylis, F.D.; Catalona, W.J.; Makarov, D.V. Time Trends and Variation in the Use of Active Surveillance for Management of Low-risk Prostate Cancer in the US. *JAMA Netw. Open* **2023**, *6*, e231439. [CrossRef] [PubMed]
11. Spellman, A.A.; Golla, V.; Lin, L.; Katz, A.; Chen, R.C.; Zullig, L.L. Long-Term Trends in Decisional Regret Among Men with Localized Prostate Cancer. *JU Open Plus* **2024**, *2*, e00027. [CrossRef]
12. Wallis, C.J.D.; Zhao, Z.; Huang, L.-C.; Penson, D.F.; Koyama, T.; Kaplan, S.H.; Greenfield, S.; Luckenbaugh, A.N.; Klaassen, Z.; Conwill, R.; et al. Association of Treatment Modality, Functional Outcomes, and Baseline Characteristics With Treatment-Related Regret Among Men With Localized Prostate Cancer. *JAMA Oncol.* **2022**, *8*, 50–59. [CrossRef] [PubMed]
13. Leslie, S.; Soon-Sutton, W.; Skelton, W. Prostate Cancer. In *StatPearls*; StatPearls Publishing: Treasure Island, FL, USA, 2024.
14. Gordetsky, J.B.; Saylor, B.; Bae, S.; Nix, J.W.; Rais-Bahrami, S. Prostate cancer management choices in patients undergoing multiparametric magnetic resonance imaging/ultrasound fusion biopsy compared to systematic biopsy. *Urol. Oncol.* **2018**, *36*, 241.e7–241.e13. [CrossRef]
15. Dix, D.B.; McDonald, A.M.; Gordetsky, J.B.; Nix, J.W.; Thomas, J.V.; Rais-Bahrami, S. How Would MRI-targeted Prostate Biopsy Alter Radiation Therapy Approaches in Treating Prostate Cancer? *Urology* **2018**, *122*, 139–146. [CrossRef] [PubMed]
16. Gordetsky, J.B.; Schultz, L.; Porter, K.K.; Nix, J.W.; Thomas, J.V.; Del Carmen Rodriguez Pena, M.; Rais-Bahrami, S. Defining the optimal method for reporting prostate cancer grade and tumor extent on magnetic resonance/ultrasound fusion-targeted biopsies. *Hum. Pathol.* **2018**, *76*, 68–75. [CrossRef]
17. Sankineni, S.; Wood, B.J.; Rais-Bahrami, S.; Walton Diaz, A.; Hoang, A.N.; Pinto, P.A.; Choyke, P.L.; Türkbey, B. Image-guided focal therapy for prostate cancer. *Diagn. Interv. Radiol. Ank. Turk.* **2014**, *20*, 492–497. [CrossRef]
18. Deivasigamani, S.; Kotamarti, S.; Rastinehad, A.R.; Salas, R.S.; de la Rosette, J.J.M.C.H.; Lepor, H.; Pinto, P.; Ahmed, H.U.; Gill, I.; Klotz, L.; et al. Primary Whole-gland Ablation for the Treatment of Clinically Localized Prostate Cancer: A Focal Therapy Society Best Practice Statement. *Eur. Urol.* **2023**, *84*, 547–560. [CrossRef]
19. Ayerra Perez, H.; Barba Abad, J.F.; Extramiana Cameno, J. An Update on Focal Therapy for Prostate Cancer. *Clin. Genitourin. Cancer* **2023**, *21*, 712.e1–712.e8. [CrossRef] [PubMed]
20. Guillaumier, S.; Peters, M.; Arya, M.; Afzal, N.; Charman, S.; Dudderidge, T.; Hosking-Jervis, F.; Hindley, R.G.; Lewi, H.; McCartan, N.; et al. A Multicentre Study of 5-year Outcomes Following Focal Therapy in Treating Clinically Significant Nonmetastatic Prostate Cancer. *Eur. Urol.* **2018**, *74*, 422–429. [CrossRef] [PubMed]
21. Guenther, E.; Klein, N.; Zapf, S.; Weil, S.; Schlosser, C.; Rubinsky, B.; Stehling, M.K. Prostate cancer treatment with Irreversible Electroporation (IRE): Safety, efficacy and clinical experience in 471 treatments. *PLoS ONE* **2019**, *14*, e0215093. [CrossRef] [PubMed]
22. Clavien, P.A.; Barkun, J.; de Oliveira, M.L.; Vauthey, J.N.; Dindo, D.; Schulick, R.D.; de Santibañes, E.; Pekolj, J.; Slankamenac, K.; Bassi, C.; et al. The Clavien-Dindo classification of surgical complications: Five-year experience. *Ann. Surg.* **2009**, *250*, 187–196. [CrossRef]
23. Eastham, J.A.; Auffenberg, G.B.; Barocas, D.A.; Chou, R.; Crispino, T.; Davis, J.W.; Eggener, S.; Horwitz, E.M.; Kane, C.J.; Kirkby, E.; et al. Clinically Localized Prostate Cancer: AUA/ASTRO Guideline, Part I: Introduction, Risk Assessment, Staging, and Risk-Based Management. *J. Urol.* **2022**, *208*, 10–18. [CrossRef]
24. Tracey, A.T.; Nogueira, L.M.; Alvim, R.G.; Coleman, J.A.; Murray, K.S. Focal therapy for primary and salvage prostate cancer treatment: A narrative review. *Transl. Androl. Urol.* **2021**, *10*, 3144–3154. [CrossRef] [PubMed]
25. Bomers, J.G.R.; Overduin, C.G.; Jenniskens, S.F.M.; Cornel, E.B.; van Lin, E.N.J.T.; Sedelaar, J.P.M.; Fütterer, J.J. Focal Salvage MR Imaging-Guided Cryoablation for Localized Prostate Cancer Recurrence after Radiotherapy: 12-Month Follow-up. *J. Vasc. Interv. Radiol. JVIR* **2020**, *31*, 35–41. [CrossRef]
26. Kanthabalan, A.; Peters, M.; Van Vulpen, M.; McCartan, N.; Hindley, R.G.; Emara, A.; Moore, C.M.; Arya, M.; Emberton, M.; Ahmed, H.U. Focal salvage high-intensity focused ultrasound in radiorecurrent prostate cancer. *BJU Int.* **2017**, *120*, 246–256. [CrossRef]

27. Schaeffer, E.M.; Srinivas, S.; Adra, N.; An, Y.; Barocas, D.; Bitting, R.; Bryce, A.; Chapin, B.; Cheng, H.H.; D'Amico, A.V.; et al. Prostate Cancer, Version 4.2023, NCCN Clinical Practice Guidelines in Oncology. *J. Natl. Compr. Cancer Netw. JNCCN* **2023**, *21*, 1067–1096. [CrossRef] [PubMed]
28. Javier-DesLoges, J.; Dall'Era, M.A.; Brisbane, W.; Chamie, K.; Washington, S.L.; Chandrasekar, T.; Marks, L.S.; Nguyen, H.; Daneshvar, M.; Gin, G.; et al. The state of focal therapy in the treatment of prostate cancer: The university of California collaborative (UC-Squared) consensus statement. *Prostate Cancer Prostatic Dis.* **2024**, *27*, 579–581. [CrossRef] [PubMed]
29. Mottet, N.; van den Bergh, R.C.N.; Briers, E.; Van den Broeck, T.; Cumberbatch, M.G.; De Santis, M.; Fanti, S.; Fossati, N.; Gandaglia, G.; Gillessen, S.; et al. EAU-EANM-ESTRO-ESUR-SIOG Guidelines on Prostate Cancer-2020 Update. Part 1: Screening, Diagnosis, and Local Treatment with Curative Intent. *Eur. Urol.* **2021**, *79*, 243–262. [CrossRef] [PubMed]
30. Ong, S.; Chen, K.; Grummet, J.; Yaxley, J.; Scheltema, M.J.; Stricker, P.; Tay, K.J.; Lawrentschuk, N. Guidelines of guidelines: Focal therapy for prostate cancer, is it time for consensus? *BJU Int.* **2023**, *131*, 20–31. [CrossRef]
31. Rodríguez-Sánchez, L.; Reiter, R.; Rodríguez, A.; Emberton, M.; de Reijke, T.; Compérat, E.M.; Bossi, A.; Sanchez-Salas, R. The FocAL therapy CONsensus (FALCON): Enhancing partial gland ablation for localised prostate cancer. *BJU Int.* **2024**, *134*, 50–53. [CrossRef]
32. Rodriguez-Sanchez, L.; Cathelineau, X.; de Reijke, T.M.; Stricker, P.; Emberton, M.; Lantz, A.; Miñana López, B.; Dominguez-Escrig, J.L.; Bianco, F.J.; Salomon, G.; et al. Refining partial gland ablation for localised prostate cancer: The FALCON project. *BJU Int.* **2025**, *135*, 1000–1009. [CrossRef]
33. Scheltema, M.J.; Tay, K.J.; Postema, A.W.; de Bruin, D.M.; Feller, J.; Futterer, J.J.; George, A.K.; Gupta, R.T.; Kahmann, F.; Kastner, C.; et al. Utilization of multiparametric prostate magnetic resonance imaging in clinical practice and focal therapy: Report from a Delphi consensus project. *World J. Urol.* **2017**, *35*, 695–701. [CrossRef]
34. Gordetsky, J.; Rais-Bahrami, S.; Epstein, J.I. Pathological Findings in Multiparametric Magnetic Resonance Imaging/Ultrasound Fusion-guided Biopsy: Relation to Prostate Cancer Focal Therapy. *Urology* **2017**, *105*, 18–23. [CrossRef]
35. Flegar, L.; Zacharis, A.; Aksoy, C.; Heers, H.; Derigs, M.; Eisenmenger, N.; Borkowetz, A.; Groeben, C.; Huber, J. Alternative- and focal therapy trends for prostate cancer: A total population analysis of in-patient treatments in Germany from 2006 to 2019. *World J. Urol.* **2022**, *40*, 1645–1652. [CrossRef] [PubMed]
36. Bozzini, G.; Colin, P.; Nevoux, P.; Villers, A.; Mordon, S.; Betrouni, N. Focal Therapy of prostate cancer: Energies and procedures. *Urol. Oncol. Semin. Orig. Investig.* **2013**, *31*, 155–167. [CrossRef] [PubMed]
37. Mearini, L.; Porena, M. Pros and cons of focal therapy for localised prostate cancer. *Prostate Cancer* **2011**, *2011*, 584784. [CrossRef]
38. Tay, K.J.; Fong, K.Y.; Stabile, A.; Dominguez-Escrig, J.L.; Ukimura, O.; Rodriguez-Sanchez, L.; Blana, A.; Becher, E.; Laguna, M.P. Established focal therapy-HIFU, IRE, or cryotherapy-where are we now?—A systematic review and meta-analysis. *Prostate Cancer Prostatic Dis.* **2024**. [CrossRef] [PubMed]
39. Hopstaken, J.S.; Bomers, J.G.R.; Sedelaar, M.J.P.; Valerio, M.; Fütterer, J.J.; Rovers, M.M. An Updated Systematic Review on Focal Therapy in Localized Prostate Cancer: What Has Changed over the Past 5 Years? *Eur. Urol.* **2022**, *81*, 5–33. [CrossRef] [PubMed]
40. van Velthoven, R.; Aoun, F.; Marcelis, Q.; Albisinni, S.; Zanaty, M.; Lemort, M.; Peltier, A.; Limani, K. A prospective clinical trial of HIFU hemiablation for clinically localized prostate cancer. *Prostate Cancer Prostatic Dis.* **2016**, *19*, 79–83. [CrossRef] [PubMed]
41. Arnouil, N.; Gelet, A.; Matillon, X.; Rouviere, O.; Colombel, M.; Ruffion, A.; Mège-Lechevallier, F.; Subtil, F.; Badet, L.; Crouzet, S. [Focal HIFU vs robot-assisted total prostatectomy: Functionnal and oncologic outcomes at one year]. *Prog. Urol.* **2018**, *28*, 603–610. [CrossRef]
42. Nahar, B.; Bhat, A.; Reis, I.M.; Soodana-Prakash, N.; Becerra, M.F.; Lopategui, D.; Venkatramani, V.; Patel, R.; Madhusoodanan, V.; Kryvenko, O.N.; et al. Prospective Evaluation of Focal High Intensity Focused Ultrasound for Localized Prostate Cancer. *J. Urol.* **2020**, *204*, 483–489. [CrossRef] [PubMed]
43. Mendez, M.H.; Passoni, N.M.; Pow-Sang, J.; Jones, J.S.; Polascik, T.J. Comparison of Outcomes Between Preoperatively Potent Men Treated with Focal Versus Whole Gland Cryotherapy in a Matched Population. *J. Endourol.* **2015**, *29*, 1193–1198. [CrossRef] [PubMed]
44. Tan, Y.G.; Law, Y.M.; Ngo, N.T.; Khor, L.Y.; Tan, P.H.; Ong, E.H.W.; Yuen, J.S.P.; Ho, H.S.S.; Tuan, J.K.L.; Kanesvaran, R.; et al. Patient-reported functional outcomes and oncological control after primary focal cryotherapy for clinically significant prostate cancer: A Phase II mandatory biopsy-monitored study. *Prostate* **2023**, *83*, 781–791. [CrossRef] [PubMed]
45. Rastinehad, A.; Deivasigamani, S.; Schwartz, M.J.; Ward, J.F.; George, A.; Sidana, A.; Becher, E.; Katz, A.E.; Sanchez-Salas, R.; Polascik, T.J. MP25-16 FOCAL CRYOTHERAPY FOR LOCALIZED PROSTATE CANCER: INITIAL REPORT FROM THE INTERNATIONAL FOCAL THERAPY SOCIETY (FTS) REGISTRY. *J. Urol.* **2024**, *211*, e410. [CrossRef]
46. Xia, Z.-Y.; Yang, J.; Xiao, F.; Xu, J.-Z.; Zhong, X.-Y.; Wang, S.-G.; Xia, Q.-D. A preliminary follow-up study on irreversible electroporation therapy in older patients with prostate cancer. *Discov. Oncol.* **2025**, *16*, 278. [CrossRef]
47. Ślusarczyk, A.; Gurwin, A.; Barnaś, A.; Ismail, H.; Miszczyk, M.; Zapała, P.; Przydacz, M.; Krajewski, W.; Antczak, A.; Życzkowski, M.; et al. Outcomes of Focal Therapy for Localized Prostate Cancer: A Systematic Review and Meta-analysis of Prospective Studies. *Eur. Urol. Oncol.* **2025**, S2588931125000392. [CrossRef] [PubMed]

48. Stabile, A.; Pellegrino, A.; Mazzone, E.; Cannoletta, D.; de Angelis, M.; Barletta, F.; Scuderi, S.; Cucchiara, V.; Gandaglia, G.; Raggi, D.; et al. Can Negative Prostate-specific Membrane Antigen Positron Emission Tomography/Computed Tomography Avoid the Need for Pelvic Lymph Node Dissection in Newly Diagnosed Prostate Cancer Patients? A Systematic Review and Meta-analysis with Backup Histology as Reference Standard. *Eur. Urol. Oncol.* **2022**, *5*, 1–17. [CrossRef] [PubMed]
49. Novara, G.; Ficarra, V.; Rosen, R.C.; Artibani, W.; Costello, A.; Eastham, J.A.; Graefen, M.; Guazzoni, G.; Shariat, S.F.; Stolzenburg, J.-U.; et al. Systematic review and meta-analysis of perioperative outcomes and complications after robot-assisted radical prostatectomy. *Eur. Urol.* **2012**, *62*, 431–452. [CrossRef]
50. Azzouzi, A.-R.; Vincendeau, S.; Barret, E.; Cicco, A.; Kleinclauss, F.; van der Poel, H.G.; Stief, C.G.; Rassweiler, J.; Salomon, G.; Solsona, E.; et al. Padeliporfin vascular-targeted photodynamic therapy versus active surveillance in men with low-risk prostate cancer (CLIN1001 PCM301): An open-label, phase 3, randomised controlled trial. *Lancet Oncol.* **2017**, *18*, 181–191. [CrossRef]
51. Gill, I.S.; Azzouzi, A.-R.; Emberton, M.; Coleman, J.A.; Coeytaux, E.; Scherz, A.; Scardino, P.T. PCM301 Study Group Randomized Trial of Partial Gland Ablation with Vascular Targeted Phototherapy versus Active Surveillance for Low Risk Prostate Cancer: Extended Followup and Analyses of Effectiveness. *J. Urol.* **2018**, *200*, 786–793. [CrossRef]
52. Labbate, C.V.; Klotz, L.; Morrow, M.; Cooperberg, M.; Esserman, L.; Eggener, S.E. Focal Therapy for Prostate Cancer: Evolutionary Parallels to Breast Cancer Treatment. *J. Urol.* **2023**, *209*, 49–57. [CrossRef]
53. Reddy, D.; van Son, M.; Peters, M.; Bertoncelli Tanaka, M.; Dudderidge, T.; Cullen, E.; Ho, C.L.T.; Hindley, R.G.; Emara, A.; McCracken, S.; et al. Focal therapy versus radical prostatectomy and external beam radiotherapy as primary treatment options for non-metastatic prostate cancer: Results of a cost-effectiveness analysis. *J. Med. Econ.* **2023**, *26*, 1099–1107. [CrossRef] [PubMed]
54. da Silva, P.A.L.; Lima, A.F.C. Direct costs of treating men with prostate cancer with High Intensity Focused Ultrasound. *Rev. Esc. Enferm. USP* **2023**, *57*, e20230132. [CrossRef] [PubMed]

Current Oncology MDPI

Article

Long-Term Patient-Reported Bowel and Urinary Quality of Life in Patients Treated with Intensity-Modulated Radiotherapy Versus Intensity-Modulated Proton Therapy for Localized Prostate Cancer

Kimberly R. Gergelis [1,†], Miao Bai [2,†], Jiasen Ma [3], David M. Routman [3], Bradley J. Stish [3], Brian J. Davis [3], Thomas M. Pisansky [3], Thomas J. Whitaker [4] and Richard Choo [3,*]

1 Department of Radiation Oncology, University of Rochester School of Medicine and Dentistry, 601 Elmwood Ave, Rochester, NY 14642, USA
2 Department of Operations and Information Management, University of Connecticut, 352 Mansfield Rd, Storrs, CT 06269, USA
3 Department of Radiation Oncology, Mayo Clinic, 200 First St SW, Rochester, MN 55905, USA
4 Department of Radiation Physics, Division of Radiation Oncology, The University of Texas MD Anderson Cancer Center, 1515 Holcombe Blvd, Houston, TX 77030, USA
* Correspondence: choo.c@mayo.edu; Tel.: +1-507-284-3551
† These authors contributed equally to this work.

Abstract: Purpose: This study aimed to compare long-term patient-reported outcomes in bowel and urinary domains between intensity-modulated radiotherapy (IMRT) and intensity-modulated proton therapy (IMPT) for localized prostate cancer. Methods and Materials: Patients with clinical T1–T2 prostate cancer receiving IMRT or IMPT at a tertiary cancer center from 2015–2018 were analyzed to determine the changes in the prospectively collected bowel function (BF), urinary irritative/obstructive symptoms (UO), and urinary incontinence (UI) domains of EPIC-26. The mean changes in EPIC-26 scores were evaluated from pretreatment to 24 months post-radiotherapy for each modality. A score change >50% of the baseline standard deviation was considered a clinically meaningful change. Results: A total of 82 patients treated with IMRT (52.2%) and 56 patients treated with IMPT (53.3%) completed the questionnaire at baseline and 24 months post-RT. There were no baseline differences in domain scores between treatment modalities. At 24 months post-radiotherapy, there was a significant and clinically meaningful decline in the BF mean score in the IMRT cohort (−4.52 (range −50, 29.17), $p = 0.003$), whereas the decline in BF score did not reach clinical relevance or significance (−1.88 (range −37.5, 50), $p = 0.046$) when accounting for the Bonferroni adjustment in the IMPT cohort. A higher proportion of patients treated with IMRT had a clinically relevant reduction in BF when compared with IMPT (47.37% vs. 25.93%, $p = 0.017$). The mean changes in the UI and UO scores of the IMRT and IMPT cohorts were neither statically significant nor clinically relevant. Conclusions: IMPT leads to a smaller decrease in BF than IMRT at 24 months post-RT, while there was no differential effect on UO and UI.

Keywords: quality of life; EPIC-26; prostate cancer; intensity-modulated radiotherapy; intensity-modulated proton therapy

1. Introduction

Treatment-related adverse effects and overall quality of life (QOL) are essential outcomes in prostate cancer treatment. Definitive prostate cancer treatments, including radical prostatectomy and radiotherapy (RT), can alter bladder, bowel, and sexual function [1]. Minimizing treatment-related adverse effects and maintaining QOL are crucial in patients' treatment choices.

Intensity-modulated RT (IMRT) and proton beam therapy (PBT) are conformal radiotherapy modalities that allow for dose escalation to the prostate while minimizing the dose delivered to adjacent normal structures. PBT has been used as a means of potentially increasing the therapeutic ratio of external beam RT for prostate cancer. Protons can lower the dose of radiation delivered to at-risk organs due to its Bragg peak dose distribution profile, and it potentially reduces radiation toxicity, compared to photons [2]. The question of whether this dosimetric advantage translates to decreased toxicity is of great interest.

As several single-institution studies of PBT for prostate cancer yielded encouraging results, two phase III studies investigating PBT versus IMRT for the treatment of prostate cancer are underway (ClinicalTrials.gov identifiers: NCT01617161, NCT04083937) [3–6]. The primary endpoint of both the Prostate Advanced Radiation Technologies Investigating Quality of Life (PARTIQoL) and Prostate Cancer Patients Treated with Alternative Radiation Oncology Strategies (PAROS) trials is to determine whether PBT is superior to IMRT in patient-reported bowel QOL. The PARTIQoL group recently presented their results in abstract form; the results demonstrated no difference between PBT or IMRT in the mean change in bowel score at 24 mo ($p = 0.836$), with both arms showing only a small, clinically non-meaningful decline from the baseline [7]. Patients treated with PBT on PARTIQoL could have received either pencil-beam scanning intensity-modulated proton therapy (IMPT) (49%) or passive scatter (51%) PBT. Approximately half of included patients received hypofractionation (51%).

Our group previously reported the effect of IMRT versus IMPT for prostate cancer on early urinary and bowel toxicity using the prospectively collected 26-item Expanded Prostate Index Composite (EPIC-26) [5]. This study demonstrated the significant and clinically meaningful worsening of bowel function (BF) and urinary obstructive (UO) symptom scores at the end of RT for patients receiving either IMRT or IMPT. The IMRT cohort experienced greater decrease in BF scores and had a higher proportion of patients with clinically meaningful reductions compared to IMPT. The IMRT group had significant and clinically meaningful worsening of BF at three months post-RT, whereas the change in the BF score of the IMPT cohort was no longer statistically significant nor clinically meaningful compared to the baseline. Changes in UO or urinary incontinence (UI) were neither significant nor clinically meaningful three months post-RT.

Late toxicity and QOL changes are also meaningful endpoints of interest to patients and providers. Comparative-effectiveness studies of conventional RT, three-dimensional conformal RT (3DCRT), IMRT, and PBT have been reported; however, these studies relied on Medicare claims as surrogates for clinical outcomes [8–12] that used conventional fractionation or passively scattered PBT [13,14]. As moderate hypofractionation is now an attractive alternative [15] and IMPT is increasingly used, we herein report the late toxicity outcomes of IMRT and IMPT using prospectively collected EPIC-26 data from patients treated with conventionally fractionated or moderately hypofractionated RT.

2. Materials and Methods

2.1. Patient Selection

Our cohort was selected using an Institutional-Review-Board-approved prospective registry of patients who received IMRT or IMPT to the prostate $\pm$ the proximal seminal vesicles for clinical stage T1–T2 N0 M0 prostate cancer at a tertiary cancer center between 2015 and 2018. Patients receiving pelvic lymph node irradiation were excluded. The included patients completed the EPIC-26 questionnaire prior to the initiation of RT, as well as 24 ± 9 months post-RT. All included patients were treated with 60 Gy in 20 fractions, 70.2 Gy in 26 fractions, or 78 Gy in 39 fractions, as these regimens were the most commonly utilized at our institution during this period. Ultrahypofractionated regimens were excluded.

2.2. Measurement of Patient-Reported QOL and Treatment Details

Patients prospectively completed the EPIC-26 questionnaire prior to RT (baseline), at the completion of RT, and at 3, 6, 12, 24, 36, and 48 months post-RT. The EPIC-26 questionnaire includes domain scores for BF, UO, UI, sexual function (SF), and hormonal function (HF). Responses within each domain are scored from 0–100, with higher scores indicating better function [16].

The primary outcomes included the change in BF, UO, and UI scores from pretreatment to 24 months post-RT. SF and HF domains were excluded as they were confounded by the use of androgen deprivation therapy (ADT).

Details of IMPT and IMRT treatment planning at our institution have been previously described [5].

2.3. Statistical Analysis

Differences in the demographics, clinical features, and baseline EPIC-26 BF, UO, and UI scores between patients treated with IMRT and those receiving IMPT were initially examined to assess whether a meaningful analysis of QOL change between the two modalities could be performed. The 24-month time point was selected to investigate late toxicity as 24 ± 9 months was identified as having the greatest number of responders. Baseline characteristics between the responders and the non-responders to the 24-month questionnaire were compared to assess whether the outcomes obtained from the responders could be generalized to the overall patient population.

The changes in BF, UO, and UI scores from baseline to 24 months post-RT were compared between patients treated with IMRT and those receiving IMPT. The statistical significance and clinical relevance of the score changes at 24 months post-RT were also assessed for IMRT and IMPT. A clinically meaningful change was defined as a score change that exceeded >50% of the standard deviation of a baseline score [17–19]. The difference in the proportion of patients with clinically meaningful changes between treatment with IMRT and IMPT was also assessed.

We examined the mean changes in EPIC-26 scores from baseline to 24 months post-RT for each RT modality to evaluate the late effects of RT on QOL. The evaluation of EPIC-26 score changes was limited to patients who completed the questionnaire both at baseline and at 24 ± 9 months post-RT.

We evaluated the independent effects of multiple variables to determine factors that significantly impacted EPIC-26 score changes over time. The examined variables included the RT modality, dose-fractionation regimen, use of a rectal hydrogel spacer, baseline EPIC-26 scores for BF, UO, and UI domains, age, baseline prostate-specific antigen (PSA), Gleason score, T stage, and the receipt of ADT. Due to the small number of non-White patients, race was excluded from this analysis. Stepwise backward/forward variable selections were conducted for the model construction based on the Akaike Information Criterion (AIC). Only variables with statistical significance were tabulated.

A two-sided Wilcoxon rank–sum test, a Wilcoxon signed-rank sum test, Fisher's exact test, and a *t*-test were used for the testing of statistical hypotheses, with $p < 0.05$ considered statistically significant unless specified otherwise. For analyses involving multiple pairwise comparisons, $p < 0.017$ was considered statistically significant to account for Bonferroni correction.

3. Results

3.1. Baseline Demographics and EPIC-26 Questionnaire Completion

A total of 157 patients treated with IMRT and 105 patients treated with IMPT completed the baseline pre-RT EPIC-26 questionnaire. Of those, 82 patients treated with IMRT (52.2%), and 56 patients treated with IMPT (53.3%) also completed the questionnaire at 24 months post-RT, and these patients comprised our study cohort. There were no statistical differences between the responders and non-responders with respect to age, baseline PSA, Gleason score, T stage, dose-fractionation regimen, the proportion of patients with hydrogel spacer (40% vs. 43%), the proportion of patients receiving androgen deprivation therapy (75% vs. 75%), baseline BF score (93.3 vs. 93.5), baseline UI score (88.2 vs. 87.7), or baseline UO score (85.3 vs. 87.6).

Table 1 describes the patient demographics and treatment characteristics of the IMRT and IMPT cohorts. There were no differences between the IMRT and IMPT cohorts with respect to race, mean age, mean pre-RT serum prostate-specific antigen (PSA), Gleason score, PSA distribution, or the proportion of patients receiving hydrogel spacer. IMPT patients were more likely to have T2 disease than those receiving IMRT (69.6% vs. 51.2%, $p = 0.04$). There was no difference in the proportion of patients receiving each dose-fractionation regimen between IMRT and IMPT (42.7% vs. 25.0% for 60 Gy in 20 fractions; 47.6% vs. 64.3% for 70.2 Gy in 26 fractions; 9.8% vs. 10.7% for 78 Gy in 39 fractions, respectively).

Table 1. Baseline characteristics of the IMRT cohort vs. the IMPT cohort.

Characteristics	IMRT (n = 82)	IMPT (n = 56)	*p*-Value *
Age			
Mean (range), year	70.9 (55–84)	70.7 (52–88)	0.77
Age group, n (%)			0.95
<70	33 (40.2%)	21 (37.5%)	
70–79	46 (56.1%)	33 (58.9%)	
≥80	3 (3.7%)	2 (3.6%)	
Race			
Race, n (%)			1.00
White	77 (93.9%)	53 (94.6%)	
Others	3 (3.7%)	2 (3.6%)	
Missing	2 (2.4%)	1 (1.8%)	
Pre-RT PSA			
Mean (range, ng/mL)	7.8 (0.2–39.4)	7.5 (0.2–23.2)	0.64
PSA level, n (%)			0.30
<4	25 (30.5%)	11 (19.6%)	
4–10	40 (48.8%)	34 (60.7%)	
>10	17 (20.7%)	11 (19.6%)	
Gleason score			
Group, n (%)			0.63
≤7	68 (82.9%)	49 (87.5%)	
>7	14 (17.1%)	7 (12.5%)	

Table 1. *Cont.*

Characteristics	IMRT (n = 82)	IMPT (n = 56)	*p*-Value *
T stage			
Group, n (%)			0.04
T1	40 (48.8%)	17 (30.4%)	
T2	42 (51.2%)	39 (69.6%)	
Dose-fractionation regimen			
n (%)			0.10
60 Gy/20 fractions	35 (42.7%)	14 (25.0%)	
70.2 Gy/26 fractions	39 (47.6%)	36 (64.3%)	
78 Gy/39 fractions	8 (9.8%)	6 (10.7%)	
Hydrogel spacer			
Treated with hydrogel spacer, n (%)	35 (42.7%)	20 (35.7%)	0.48
Androgen deprivation therapy (ADT)			
Treated with ADT, n (%)	64 (78.1%)	40 (71.4%)	0.42
Baseline bowel score			
Mean (range)	94.0 (62.5–100)	92.3 (50–100)	0.98
Standard deviation	8.3	12.6	
Missing	3	1	
Baseline urinary incontinence score			
Mean (range)	87.7 (22.8–99.5)	88.9 (39.3–99.5)	0.49
Standard deviation	16.7	15.8	
Missing	0	1	
Baseline urinary irritative/obstructive score			
Mean (range)	85.8 (43.8–100)	84.4 (50–100)	0.50
Standard deviation	12.6	12.6	
Missing	0	5	

* *p*-values were derived from Wilcoxon rank–sum test for continuous variables, and Fisher's exact test for categorical variables. *p*-values reflect whether the means or the distributions were different between the two cohorts. $p < 0.05$ is considered significant. IMRT: Intensity Modulated Radiation Therapy. IMPT: Intensity Modulated Proton Therapy. Pre-RT PSA: Pre-radiotherapy prostate-specific antigen. T stage: Tumor stage. Gy: Gray. ADT: Androgen deprivation therapy

3.2. Changes in the BF, UO and UI Scores Between the IMRT and IMPT Cohorts

There were no statistically significant differences in the baseline BF, UO, and UI domain scores between the IMRT and IMPT cohorts (Table 1).

In the IMRT cohort, there was a clinically relevant and significant decline in the BF mean score from baseline to 24 months post-RT ($p = 0.003$) (Table 2). In contrast, the decline in the BF mean score in the IMPT cohort was less pronounced and did not reach statistical significance when accounting for the Bonferroni adjustment ($p = 0.046$). Furthermore, its decline was not a clinically relevant reduction. The mean changes in the UI and UO scores of the IMRT and IMPT cohorts were neither statistically significant nor clinically relevant.

Table 2. Score changes and their clinical relevance for each treatment modality.

EPIC-26 Domain	Radiation Modality	No. of Respondents (%)	Mean Score Change From Baseline (Range)	p *	Clinically Relevant Change? (Y/N) **
Bowel function	IMRT	76 (92.7%)	−4.52 (−50, 29.17)	0.003	Y
	IMPT	54 (96.4%)	−1.88 (−37.5, 50)	0.046	N
Urinary incontinence	IMRT	67 (81.7%)	−2.61 (−32.75, 27.5)	0.79	N
	IMPT	51 (91.1%)	−0.80 (−39, 40)	0.75	N
Urinary irritative/obstructive	IMRT	76 (92.7%)	−0.58 (−50, 25)	0.76	N
	IMPT	51 (91.1%)	1.84 (−37.5, 43.75)	0.41	N

* p-values were derived from a Wilcoxon signed-rank–sum test and reflect whether late scores were different from baseline score. $p < 0.017$ is considered significant to account for the Bonferroni adjustment. ** When a score change exceeds > 50% of the standard deviation of baseline score, it is considered clinically relevant. IMPT: Intensity Modulated Proton Therapy. IMRT: Intensity Modulated Radiation Therapy. EPIC-26: 26-item Expanded Prostate Index Composite. Y: Yes. N: No.

A higher proportion of patients treated with IMRT had a clinically relevant reduction in BF when compared with IMPT (47.4% vs. 25.9%, $p = 0.017$), which approached significance. There was no difference in the proportion of patients with clinically relevant reductions in UI ($p = 0.82$) or UO ($p = 0.36$) scores between IMRT and IMPT (Table 3).

Table 3. Comparison of the proportions of patients with clinically relevant changes between the IMRT cohort and the IMPT cohort.

EPIC-26 Domain	Radiation Modality	Patients with Clinically Relevant Reduction (%)	p *
Bowel			
	IMRT	36 (47.4%)	0.017
	IMPT	14 (25.9%)	
Urinary Incontinence			
	IMRT	15 (22.4%)	0.82
	IMPT	10 (19.6%)	
Urinary Irritative/Obstructive			
	IMRT	12 (15.8%)	0.36
	IMPT	12 (23.5%)	

* p-values derived from Fisher's exact test. p-values test whether the difference in the proportion of patients experiencing clinically relevant reduction is statistically significant between two modalities. $p < 0.017$ is considered significant to account for the Bonferroni adjustment. IMPT: Intensity Modulated Proton Therapy. IMRT: Intensity Modulated Radiation Therapy. EPIC-26: 26-item Expanded Prostate Index Composite

The mean score changes in BF, UO, and UI domains from baseline to 24 months post-RT of the IMRT and IMPT cohorts are described and compared in Table 4. The mean BF and UI scores declined in both cohorts. The mean score of the UO domain improved from baseline in the IMPT cohort, whereas it declined in the IMRT cohort. Although the mean score decline in the BF domain was less in the IMPT cohort (−1.88) than in the IMRT cohort (−4.52), the difference in the mean score decline between the two cohorts was not statistically significant. There were also no statistical differences in the mean score changes in UI and UO domains when comparing the IMRT and IMPT cohorts.

Table 4. Comparison of score changes between the IMRT cohort and IMPT cohort.

EPIC-26 Domain	Radiation Modality	Late Response	
		Mean Change from Baseline	p *
Bowel			
	IMRT	−4.52	0.69
	IMPT	−1.88	
Urinary Incontinence			
	IMRT	−2.61	0.55
	IMPT	−0.80	
Urinary Irritative/Obstructive			
	IMRT	−0.58	0.64
	IMPT	1.84	

* p-values were derived from a Wilcoxon rank–sum test. p-values reflect whether score changes were different between two treatment cohorts. $p < 0.017$ is considered significant to account for the Bonferroni correction. IMPT: Intensity Modulated Proton Therapy IMRT: Intensity Modulated Radiation Therapy EPIC-26: 26-item Expanded Prostate Index Composite

3.3. *Variables Associated with Domain Score Changes*

The variables associated with the domain score changes from baseline to 24 months post-RT are summarized in Table 5. A greater reduction in the BF domain for all patients was associated with a higher baseline BF score (i.e., fewer bowel symptoms) ($p < 0.001$) and a lower baseline UO score (i.e., more irritative/obstructive symptoms) ($p = 0.01$). A greater reduction in the UO domain was associated with a higher baseline UO score (i.e., fewer irritative/obstructive symptoms) ($p \leq 0.001$). A greater reduction in the UI domain was associated with a higher baseline UI score (i.e., less urinary incontinence) ($p < 0.001$). The domain score changes were not associated with the radiation modality, dose-fractionation regimens, or use of a hydrogel spacer.

Table 5. Factors associated with late changes in each domain of the EPIC-26 score.

EPIC-26 Domain	Independent Variable	Coefficient	p-Value *
Bowel	Baseline BF score	−0.9	<0.001
	Baseline UO score	0.2	0.01
Urinary incontinence	Baseline UI score	−0.4	<0.001
Urinary irritative/obstructive	Baseline UO score	−0.7	<0.001

* Multivariable linear regression was used to identify factors that were statistically significantly associated with changes in the scores. p-values test the individual covariate effect. $p < 0.05$ is considered significant. Variables included in the regression models were the type of radiation modality (IMPT vs. IMRT), the dose fractionation regimen utilized (60 Gy/20 fraction vs. 70.2 Gy/26 fraction vs. 78 Gy/39 fraction), the use of a hydrogel spacer (yes vs. no), baseline BF, UO, and UI scores, age, PSA, the Gleason score, the T stage, and the use of ADT. We excluded race from this analysis because of the small number of non-Caucasian patients. Stepwise backward/forward variable selections were conducted for the model construction based on the Akaike Information Criterion (AIC). Only those variables found to be statistically significant are tabulated. EPIC-26: 26-item Expanded Prostate Index Composite. BF: Bowel function symptom score. UO: Urinary irritative/obstructive symptom score. UI: Urinary incontinence symptom score

4. Discussion

Our group previously reported early toxicity differences between IMRT and IMPT prostate RT, showing that the IMRT cohort experienced greater decrease in BF at the end of RT, and that a higher proportion of patients have a clinically meaningful reduction compared with IMPT. The IMRT group exhibited a significant and clinically meaningful worsening of BF at three months following the completion of RT, whereas the change in BF score of the IMPT cohort was neither statistically significant nor clinically meaningful compared to the baseline. At three months following the completion of RT, there were no statistically significant nor clinically meaningful changes in UO or UI. As early toxicity generally improves with time, an evaluation of late effects is an important addition to the toxicity profile of any treatment, which prompted this study.

With continued follow up, we found that patients treated with IMRT had a significant and clinically meaningful decrease in BF two years after completing treatment, whereas IMPT- treated patients did not. In addition, the percentage of patients with a clinically relevant reduction in BF score was greater with IMRT than with IMPT, and this approached significance. However, in our multivariable linear regression analysis, we did not identify an association between the treatment modality and a change in the BF domain score from baseline to 24 months post-RT. Only better baseline BF and worse baseline UO scores were associated with decline in BF score at 24 months. This lack of an association between the treatment modality and changes in the BF domain score according to the multivariate analysis is possibly due to the small number of patients included in this study, with response rates at 24 months of 52.2% and 53.3% for IMRT and IMPT, respectively. That is, our sample size was insufficient to detect a difference, if one existed. There were no significant or clinically meaningful differences in UI or UO domain scores at 24 months between patients treated with IMRT or IMPT.

Hoppe et al. completed a similar study at the University of Florida [13] and, similarly, found that only BF scores met the minimally detectable difference from baseline at six months, one year, and two years for IMRT, and at one year and two years for PBT. In their study, more patients treated with IMRT had a minimally detectable difference in BF score from baseline at six months ($p = 0.002$); however, there was no difference between modalities at one and two years. This differs from our study, because the patients treated with IMRT at our institution reported a clinically meaningful reduction in BF at two years compared to patients treated with IMPT. However, our studies have differences that may affect the outcomes and interpretation of results. Hoppe et al. compared a group treated with conventionally fractionated (1.8 Gy or 2.0 Gy per fraction) passive scatter PBT at their center with IMRT patients treated at nine other centers during an earlier timeframe. In contrast, our patients mainly received moderately hypofractionated (2.7 Gy or 3.0 Gy per fraction) RT at only one institution. Our report may be more germane to contemporary practice, because hypofractionated RT has become a standard of care for organ-confined prostate carcinoma. The patients in our study were treated with pencil-beam IMPT, rather than passive scatter, which is a newer and more conformal technology.

A matched-pair analysis conducted by Dutz et al. compared patient-reported early and late toxicities using the EORTC-QLQ-C30/PR25, dosimetric parameters, and QOL between conventionally fractionated passive scatter PBT and IMRT in prostate cancer patients [20]. Their study identified significantly lower late urinary urgency in patients receiving PBT, and it also found that late grade ≥ 2 GU toxicities were associated with the relative volume of the anterior bladder wall receiving 70 Gy and the entire bladder receiving 60 Gy. Their study is limited by the use of passive scatter and patient-reported QOL only for one year.

The University of Washington reported their experience [21] of patient-reported QOL with conventionally fractioned IMPT for prostate cancer and found that EPIC bowel domain declined at one-year post-treatment compared to baseline with no further decline over time; however, the IMPT cohort was not compared to an IMRT cohort. They also had a more heterogeneous study cohort than ours, as some of their patients also received pelvic nodal

RT. Pugh et al. conducted a similar study [22] investigating the QOL of patients receiving conventionally fractionated passive scatter PBT or IMPT for prostate cancer; similarly, they found a clinically significant decrement in bowel QOL over time. However, there was no IMRT comparative cohort in their study.

Bulman et al. investigated the rectal dose and changes in bowel-related QOL in patients treated with IMPT and correlated QOL to dosimetric parameters [23]. Their study examined a heterogeneous cohort, including patients treated with conventional, moderate hypofractionation, as well as ultrahypofractionation. The BF domain score declined from baseline to the end of treatment and at 12 months; however, this study did not investigate whether it was a clinically meaningful decline. They found that rectal BED D25 (Gy) $\geq$23% was significantly associated with decline.

The Phase III PARTIQoL study recently presented results in abstract form; these results demonstrated no difference between PBT or IMRT in the mean change in the bowel score at 24 months ($p = 0.836$), with both arms showing only small, clinically non-meaningful decline from baseline [6,7]. This study included a large number of patients treated with PBT and IMRT (n = 226 and n = 224, respectively). Like our cohort, participants received treatment to the prostate and proximal seminal vesicles; pelvic nodal RT was not performed. Our results differ from those of the PARTIQoL study; in our cohort, patients treated with IMRT had a significant and clinically meaningful decrement in BF two years after completing treatment, whereas the IMPT- treated patients did not. Both IMPT (49%) and passive scatter (51%) techniques were utilized in the PBT cohort of PARTIQoL, whereas all patients in our PBT cohort received IMPT. It is possible that the PBT technique or bowel and/or rectum dosimetry may account for this discrepancy. It is also possible that we detected differences in bowel QOL by chance.

Our study has multiple limitations. First, our study was not designed as a randomized clinical trial. Thus, it does not offer a definitive comparison between IMRT and IMPT, and there may be selection bias and unknown factors affecting treatment outcomes and the type of treatment modality a patient received. Second, our evaluation of QOL change was limited to a single post-RT timepoint, because not every patient answered the EPIC-26 surveys at each specified time point. Treatment-related QOL may change over time, and we were not able to capture this information or to present the QOL data as a continuum. Third, we had a relatively small number of patients, and this may introduce some uncertainty that a larger study cohort would not face. Thus, the results of our study need to be interpreted with caution. Fourth, we did not examine whether a potential benefit of IMPT in BF outcome justifies the additional cost of proton therapy. Lastly, although our study suggests that patients treated with IMPT experience lower rates of late BF decline, we did not correlate this with the dose-volume histogram (DVH) parameters used in planning RT.

5. Conclusions

Most previously published reports of patients treated with IMRT and PBT for localized prostate cancer have found a decline in BF QOL after RT. Our study provides a single institution's comparative analysis between IMRT and IMPT for BF, UO, and UI changes at 24 months post-RT using prospectively collected EPIC-26 data. In our experience, IMPT continued to show less of a decrease in BF than IMRT at 24 months post-RT, whereas there was no differential effect on UO and UI between treatment modalities. Further work, including dosimetric studies correlating QOL with DVH parameters and randomized trials, are needed to determine whether there is a clinically meaningful difference in tumor control, RT adverse effects, and QOL changes between IMRT and IMPT.

Author Contributions: Conceptualization, K.R.G., R.C., T.J.W., D.M.R. and M.B.; methodology, K.R.G., M.B., J.M., D.M.R., T.J.W. and R.C.; validation, K.R.G., M.B., T.J.W. and R.C.; formal analysis, M.B.; investigation, K.R.G., M.B., T.J.W. and R.C.; data curation, T.J.W.; writing—original draft preparation, K.R.G. and M.B.; writing—review and editing, K.R.G., D.M.R., B.J.S., B.J.D., T.M.P., T.J.W. and R.C.; visualization, K.R.G. and M.B.; supervision, R.C. All authors have read and agreed to the published version of the manuscript.

Funding: This research received no external funding.

Institutional Review Board Statement: The study was conducted in accordance with the Declaration of Helsinki and approved by the Institutional Review Board (or Ethics Committee) of Mayo Clinic (18-009974) on 23 November 2018.

Informed Consent Statement: Patient consent was waived due to the retrospective nature of this study.

Data Availability Statement: The data presented in this study are available on request from the corresponding author due to institutional requirements regarding data sharing.

Conflicts of Interest: Davis reports receiving personal fees and other from Boston Scientific, Inc. during the course of the study; other from Pfizer, Inc., other from the American Brachytherapy Society, and nonfinancial support from the American Board of Radiology outside the submitted work. The remaining authors declare no conflicts of interest.

References

1. Donovan, J.L.; Hamdy, F.C.; Lane, J.A.; Mason, M.; Metcalfe, C.; Walsh, E.; Blazeby, J.M.; Peters, T.J.; Holding, P.; Bonnington, S.; et al. Patient-Reported Outcomes after Monitoring, Surgery, or Radiotherapy for Prostate Cancer. *N. Engl. J. Med.* **2016**, *375*, 1425–1437.
2. Whitaker, T.J.; Routman, D.M.; Schultz, H.; Harmsen, W.S.; Corbin, K.S.; Wong, W.W.; Choo, R. IMPT versus VMAT for Pelvic Nodal Irradiation in Prostate Cancer: A Dosimetric Comparison. *Int. J. Part. Ther.* **2019**, *5*, 11–23. [CrossRef] [PubMed]
3. Bryant, C.; Smith, T.L.; Henderson, R.H.; Hoppe, B.S.; Mendenhall, W.M.; Nichols, R.C.; Morris, C.G.; Williams, C.R.; Su, Z.; Li, Z.; et al. Five-Year Biochemical Results, Toxicity, and Patient-Reported Quality of Life After Delivery of Dose-Escalated Image Guided Proton Therapy for Prostate Cancer. *Int. J. Radiat. Oncol. Biol. Phys.* **2016**, *95*, 422–434. [PubMed]
4. Takagi, M.; Demizu, Y.; Terashima, K.; Fujii, O.; Jin, D.; Niwa, Y.; Daimon, T.; Murakami, M.; Fuwa, N.; Okimoto, T. Long-term outcomes in patients treated with proton therapy for localized prostate cancer. *Cancer Med.* **2017**, *6*, 2234–2243. [PubMed]
5. Bai, M.; Gergelis, K.R.; Sir, M.; Whitaker, T.J.; Routman, D.M.; Stish, B.J.; Davis, B.J.; Pisansky, T.M.; Choo, R. Comparing bowel and urinary domains of patient-reported quality of life at the end of and 3 months post radiotherapy between intensity-modulated radiotherapy and proton beam therapy for clinically localized prostate cancer. *Cancer Med.* **2020**, *9*, 7925–7934.
6. Wisdom, A.J.; Yeap, B.Y.; Michalski, J.M.; Horick, N.K.; Zietman, A.L.; Christodouleas, J.P.; Kamran, S.C.; Parikh, R.R.; Vapiwala, N.; Mihalcik, S.; et al. Setting the Stage: Feasibility and Baseline Characteristics in the PARTIQoL Trial Comparing Proton Therapy Versus Intensity Modulated Radiation Therapy for Localized Prostate Cancer. *Int. J. Radiat. Oncol. Biol. Phys.* **2025**, *121*, 741–751.
7. Efstathiou, J.A.; Yeap, B.Y.; Michalski, J.M.; Horick, N.; Zietman, A.L.; Christodouleas, J.P.; Kamran, S.C.; Parikh, R.R.; Vapiwala, N.; Mihalcik, S.A.; et al. Prostate Advanced Radiation Technologies Investigating Quality of Life (PARTIQoL): Phase III Randomized Clinical Trial of Proton Therapy vs. IMRT for Localized Prostate Cancer. *Int. J. Radiat. Oncol. Biol. Phys.* **2024**, *120*, S1. [CrossRef]
8. Bekelman, J.E.; Mitra, N.; Efstathiou, J.; Liao, K.; Sunderland, R.; Yeboa, D.N.; Armstrong, K. Outcomes after intensity-modulated versus conformal radiotherapy in older men with nonmetastatic prostate cancer. *Int. J. Radiat. Oncol. Biol. Phys.* **2011**, *81*, e325–e334. [CrossRef]
9. Sheets, N.C.; Goldin, G.H.; Meyer, A.M.; Wu, Y.; Chang, Y.; Stürmer, T.; Holmes, J.A.; Reeve, B.B.; Godley, P.A.; Carpenter, W.R.; et al. Intensity-modulated radiation therapy, proton therapy, or conformal radiation therapy and morbidity and disease control in localized prostate cancer. *JAMA* **2012**, *307*, 1611–1620.
10. Kim, S.; Shen, S.; Moore, D.F.; Shih, W.; Lin, Y.; Li, H.; Dolan, M.; Shao, Y.H.; Lu-Yao, G.L. Late gastrointestinal toxicities following radiation therapy for prostate cancer. *Eur. Urol.* **2011**, *60*, 908–916. [CrossRef]
11. Yu, J.B.; Soulos, P.R.; Herrin, J.; Cramer, L.D.; Potosky, A.L.; Roberts, K.B.; Gross, C.P. Proton versus intensity-modulated radiotherapy for prostate cancer: Patterns of care and early toxicity. *J. Natl. Cancer Inst.* **2013**, *105*, 25–32. [PubMed]
12. Yu, J.B.; DeStephano, D.M.; Jeffers, B.; Horowitz, D.P.; Soulos, P.R.; Gross, C.P.; Cheng, S.K. Updated Analysis of Comparative Toxicity of Proton and Photon Radiation for Prostate Cancer. *J. Clin. Oncol.* **2024**, *42*, 1943–1952.

13. Hoppe, B.S.; Michalski, J.M.; Mendenhall, N.P.; Morris, C.G.; Henderson, R.H.; Nichols, R.C.; Mendenhall, W.M.; Williams, C.R.; Regan, M.M.; Chipman, J.J.; et al. Comparative effectiveness study of patient-reported outcomes after proton therapy or intensity-modulated radiotherapy for prostate cancer. *Cancer* **2014**, *120*, 1076–1082. [PubMed]
14. Gray, P.J.; Paly, J.J.; Yeap, B.Y.; Sanda, M.G.; Sandler, H.M.; Michalski, J.M.; Talcott, J.A.; Coen, J.J.; Hamstra, D.A.; Shipley, W.U.; et al. Patient-reported outcomes after 3-dimensional conformal, intensity-modulated, or proton beam radiotherapy for localized prostate cancer. *Cancer* **2013**, *119*, 1729–1735.
15. NCCN Clinical Practice Guidelines in Oncology (NCCN Guidelines®) for Prostate Cancer V.1.2025. © National Comprehensive Cancer Network, Inc., 2024. All Rights Reserved. Available online: https://www.nccn.org/guidelines/guidelines-detail?category=1&id=1459 (accessed on 1 April 2025).
16. Szymanski, K.M.; Wei, J.T.; Dunn, R.L.; Sanda, M.G. Development and validation of an abbreviated version of the expanded prostate cancer index composite instrument for measuring health-related quality of life among prostate cancer survivors. *Urology* **2010**, *76*, 1245–1250. [PubMed]
17. Norman, G.R.; Sloan, J.A.; Wyrwich, K.W. Interpretation of changes in health-related quality of life: The remarkable universality of half a standard deviation. *Med. Care* **2003**, *41*, 582–592.
18. Bruner, D.W.; Pugh, S.L.; Lee, W.R.; Hall, W.A.; Dignam, J.J.; Low, D.; Swanson, G.P.; Shah, A.B.; Malone, S.; Michalski, J.M.; et al. Quality of Life in Patients With Low-Risk Prostate Cancer Treated With Hypofractionated vs Conventional Radiotherapy: A Phase 3 Randomized Clinical Trial. *JAMA Oncol.* **2019**, *5*, 664–670.
19. Sanda, M.G.; Dunn, R.L.; Michalski, J.; Sandler, H.M.; Northouse, L.; Hembroff, L.; Lin, X.; Greenfield, T.K.; Litwin, M.S.; Saigal, C.S.; et al. Quality of life and satisfaction with outcome among prostate-cancer survivors. *N. Engl. J. Med.* **2008**, *358*, 1250–1261.
20. Dutz, A.; Agolli, L.; Baumann, M.; Troost, E.G.C.; Krause, M.; Hölscher, T.; Löck, S. Early and late side effects, dosimetric parameters and quality of life after proton beam therapy and IMRT for prostate cancer: A matched-pair analysis. *Acta Oncol.* **2019**, *58*, 916–925.
21. Lee, H.J., Jr.; Macomber, M.W.; Spraker, M.B.; Bowen, S.R.; Hippe, D.S.; Fung, A.; Russell, K.J.; Laramore, G.E.; Rengan, R.; Liao, J.; et al. Early toxicity and patient reported quality-of-life in patients receiving proton therapy for localized prostate cancer: A single institutional review of prospectively recorded outcomes. *Radiat. Oncol.* **2018**, *13*, 179.
22. Pugh, T.J.; Choi, S.; Nogueras-Gonzalaez, G.M.; Nguyen, Q.N.; Mahmood, U.; Frank, S.J.; Mathai, B.; Zhu, X.R.; Sahoo, N.; Gillin, M.; et al. Proton Beam Therapy for Localized Prostate Cancer: Results from a Prospective Quality-of-Life Trial. *Int. J. Part. Ther.* **2016**, *3*, 27–36. [PubMed]
23. Bulman, G.F.; Bhangoo, R.S.; DeWees, T.A.; Petersen, M.M.; Thorpe, C.S.; Wong, W.W.; Rwigema, J.C.M.; Daniels, T.B.; Keole, S.R.; Schild, S.E.; et al. Dose-volume histogram parameters and patient-reported EPIC-Bowel domain in prostate cancer proton therapy. *Radiat. Oncol. J.* **2021**, *39*, 122–128. [PubMed]

Current Oncology | MDPI

Article

Quality of Life Longitudinal Evaluation in Prostate Cancer Patients from Radiotherapy Start to 5 Years after IMRT-IGRT

Angelo Maggio [1,*], Tiziana Rancati [2], Marco Gatti [1], Domenico Cante [3], Barbara Avuzzi [2], Cinzia Bianconi [4], Fabio Badenchini [2], Bruno Farina [5], Paolo Ferrari [6], Tommaso Giandini [2], Giuseppe Girelli [5], Valeria Landoni [7], Alessandro Magli [8], Eugenia Moretti [8], Edoardo Petrucci [3], Paolo Salmoiraghi [9], Giuseppe Sanguineti [7], Elisa Villa [9], Justyna Magdalena Waskiewicz [6], Alessia Guarneri [1], Riccardo Valdagni [2,10], Claudio Fiorino [4] and Cesare Cozzarini [4]

1. Istituto di Candiolo-FPO, IRCCS, 10060 Candiolo, Italy; marco.gatti@ircc.it (M.G.); alessia.guarneri@ircc.it (A.G.)
2. Fondazione IRCCS Istituto Nazionale dei Tumori di Milano, 20133 Milano, Italy; tiziana.rancati@istitutotumori.mi.it (T.R.); avuzzi.barbara@istitutotumori.mi.it (B.A.); fabio.badenchini@istitutotumori.mi.it (F.B.); tommaso.giandini@istitutotumori.mi.it (T.G.); riccardo.valdagni@unimi.it (R.V.)
3. Ospedale di Ivrea, A.S.L. TO4, 10015 Ivrea, Italy; dcante@aslto4.piemonte.it (D.C.); epetrucci@aslto4.piemonte.it (E.P.)
4. IRCCS Ospedale San Raffaele, 20132 Milano, Italy; bianconi.cinzia@hsr.it (C.B.); fiorino.claudio@hsr.it (C.F.); cozzarini.cesare@hsr.it (C.C.)
5. Ospedale degli Infermi, 13875 Biella, Italy; bruno.farina@aslbi.piemonte.it (B.F.); giuseppe.girelli@albi.pemont.it (G.G.)
6. Comprensorio Sanitario di Bolzano, 39100 Bolzano, Italy; paolo.ferrari@sabes.it (P.F.); justynamagdalena.waskiewicz@sabes.it (J.M.W.)
7. IRCCS Istituto Tumori Regina Elena, 00144 Roma, Italy; valeria.landoni@ifo.gov.it (V.L.); giuseppe.sanguineti@ifo.it (G.S.)
8. Ospedale di Udine, 33100 Udine, Italy; alessandro.magli@asufc.sanita.fvg.it (A.M.); eugenia.moretti@ausfc.sanita.fvg.it (E.M.)
9. Cliniche Gavazzeni-Humanitas, 24121 Bergamo, Italy; paolo.salmoiraghi@gavazzeni.it (P.S.); elisa.villa@gavazzeni.it (E.V.)
10. Department of Oncology and Hemato-Oncology, Università degli Studi di Milano, 20122 Milano, Italy

* Correspondence: maggio.angelo@gmail.com

Abstract: Purpose: The purpose of this study is to study the evolution of quality of life (QoL) in the first 5 years following Intensity-modulated radiation therapy (IMRT) for prostate cancer (PCa) and to determine possible associations with clinical/treatment data. Material and methods: Patients were enrolled in a prospective multicentre observational trial in 2010-2014 and treated with conventional (74–80 Gy, 1.8–2 Gy/fr) or moderately hypofractionated IMRT (65–75.2 Gy, 2.2–2.7 Gy/fr). QoL was evaluated by means of EORTC QLQ-C30 at baseline, at radiation therapy (RT) end, and every 6 months up to 5 years after IMRT end. Fourteen QoL dimensions were investigated separately. The longitudinal evaluation of QoL was analysed by means of Analysis of variances (ANOVA) for multiple measures. Results: A total of 391 patients with complete sets of questionnaires across 5 years were available. The longitudinal analysis showed a trend toward the significant worsening of QoL at RT end for global health, physical and role functioning, fatigue, appetite loss, diarrhoea, and pain. QoL worsening was recovered within 6 months from RT end, with the only exception being physical functioning. Based on ANOVA, the most impaired time point was RT end. QoL dimension analysis at this time indicated that acute Grade ≥ 2 gastrointestinal (GI) toxicity significantly impacted global health, physical and role functioning, fatigue, appetite loss, diarrhoea, and pain. Acute Grade ≥ 2 genitourinary (GU) toxicity resulted in lower role functioning and higher pain. Prophylactic lymph-nodal irradiation (WPRT) resulted in significantly lower QoL for global health, fatigue, appetite loss, and diarrhoea; lower pain with the use of neoadjuvant/concomitant hormonal therapy; and lower fatigue with the use of an anti-androgen. Conclusions: In this prospective, longitudinal, observational study, high radiation IMRT doses delivered for PCa led to a temporary worsening of QoL, which tended to be completely resolved at six months. Such transient worsening was mostly associated with acute GI/GU toxicity, WPRT, and higher prescription doses.

Keywords: prostate cancer; radiotherapy; EORTCQLQ-C30 questionnaire; quality of life

1. Introduction

Radiation therapy is a widely used, highly effective, therapeutic modality for the definitive treatment of locally advanced or localized prostate cancer (PCa), with or without the combination of androgen deprivation [1–6]. With the continuous improvement of clinical outcome, radiation oncologists increasingly pay attention to the possible impact of side effects on an individual's functioning, physical, and/or psychosocial domains. For this reason, patient-reported outcomes (PROs) concerning health-related quality of life (HRQoL) need to be increasingly considered in order to better investigate more subjective parameters (e.g., physical, social, or role functioning), possibly allowing for the identification of bothersome symptoms not highlighted by physician-reported toxicity. Consequently, patients' HRQoL is more and more becoming a noteworthy factor supporting the decisions regarding treatment options [7]. Donovan et al. [8] compared the subjective outcomes of 1643 men managed with active monitoring, radical prostatectomy, or external-beam radiotherapy (EBRT) for their clinically localized prostate cancer. The patient-reported HRQoL evaluated by means of questionnaires emphasized that prostatectomy had the greatest negative effect on the patients' sexual and urinary function while EBRT had only a little effect on urinary continence. Similar findings were reported by systematic reviews focused on a quality of life comparison among surgery, radiotherapy, surveille, or brachytherapy [9]. Additional studies evaluating changes in quality of life in PCa patients undergoing radiotherapy and that aimed at identifying factors that influence QoL were performed. Yucel et al. [10], evaluating 367 PCa patients treated with definitive RT, observed a transient radiation-induced deterioration of patients' HRQoL, with complete restoration by one month from radiotherapy end. Furthermore, a correlation between HRQoL and disease-specific and patient-specific factors was found.

One of the most widely used instruments to assess the QoL of cancer patients is the EORTC QLQ-C30 questionnaire [11] developed in 2001 by the European Organisation for Research and Treatment of Cancer (EORTC).

The aim of the current paper was to investigate patients' HRQoL changes in the first 5 years following intensity-modulated radiotherapy (IMRT) for prostate cancer in a large, prospectively followed multicentric cohort and to determine possible associations with clinical and treatment factors.

2. Materials and Methods

Between April 2010 and December 2014, 391 patients treated with definitive IMRT for both clinically localized or locally advanced, non-metastatic, prostate cancer were enrolled in a prospective, longitudinal, multicentre observational trial aimed at developing predictive models of both urinary toxicity and erectile dysfunction. The DUE-01 (Urinary and Erectile Disfunction after radical RT for localized prostate cancer) study was approved by the local Ethical Committee of any participating institution, and written informed consent for the inclusion in the study was obtained for each enrolled patient. The study's coordinator centre Ethics Committee Name is "IL COMITATO ETICO dell'Ospedale San Raffaele–Milano, Istituto di Ricovero e Cura a Carattere Scientifico" with approval protocol N°: DUE-01.

Detailed information about the trial was reported previously [12,13]. In short, relevant clinical, dosimetric, and patient-reported toxicity data were prospectively collected. Patients were treated at different prescription doses with conventional (74–80 Gy, 1.8–2 Gy/fr) or moderately hypofractionated IMRT (65–75.2 Gy, 2.2–2.7 Gy/fr), always with 5 fractions/week. The prescribed doses D were converted into 2 Gy equivalent doses (EQD2), according to the linear quadratic model [14] considering the formula $EQD2 = D(\alpha/\beta + d)/(\alpha/\beta + 2)$, where d is the daily dose and the α/β ratio is a measure of the fractionation sensitivity of the cells.

This value was set according to the literature-reported data [14,15] depending on the toxicity endpoint investigated.

All patients were treated supine with an empty rectum and comfortably full bladder.

Patients were treated at eight institutions, as shown in Table 1, while patients' characteristics are indicated in Table 2. Figure 1 reports how many patients completed the questionnaire at different time points.

Table 1. Number of patients grouped according to fractionation and institution.

Institution	Patients		N
	Conventional Fractionation	Moderate Hypofractionation	
1	111	21	132
2	-	76	76
3	-	12	12
4	13	12	25
5	9	21	30
6	27	28	55
7	-	32	32
8	-	29	29

Table 2. Patient characteristics. Counts (percentage in parenthesis) for categorical variables and medians (range) for continuous variables are reported.

Age (y)	71 (67–74)
BMI (kg/m^2)	26 (19-42)
PSA (ng/mL)	6.7 (0.3–277)
Gleason score:	
<7	135
=7	186
>7	40
n.a.	30
T stage:	
T1	217
T2	117
T3-4	46
TX	11
Lymph node staging	
Nx	349
N0	39
N1	3
Diabetes	63 (16%)
Cardiovascular disease	102 (26%)
Hypercholesterolemia	23 (6%)
Urological disease	23 (6%)
Anticoagulants	27 (7%)
Antidepressive	16 (4%)
TURP	39 (10%)
Previous abdominal surgery	180 (46%)
Smoke	63 (16%)
Alcohol	188 (48%)
Hormone therapy before/during RT	227 (58%)
Pelvic irradiation (Yes/No)	167 (Yes 42.7%)/224 (No 57.3%)
Hormone therapy after RT 166 (56%)	226 (58%)
Prescribed dose (Gy)	HYPO (n = 231): 70.2 (54.3–74.2) CONV (n = 160): 76 (74–83.2)
Daily dose (Gy/fr)	HYPO: 2.55 (2.2–3.8) CONV: 2.0 (1.8–2.0)
CTV volume (cc) 51 (34–66)	52 (11–180)
PTV volume (cc) 131 (93–170)	132 (28–350)

(BMI = body mass index; TURP = transurethal resection of prostate; CTV = clinical target volume; PTV = planning target volume.)

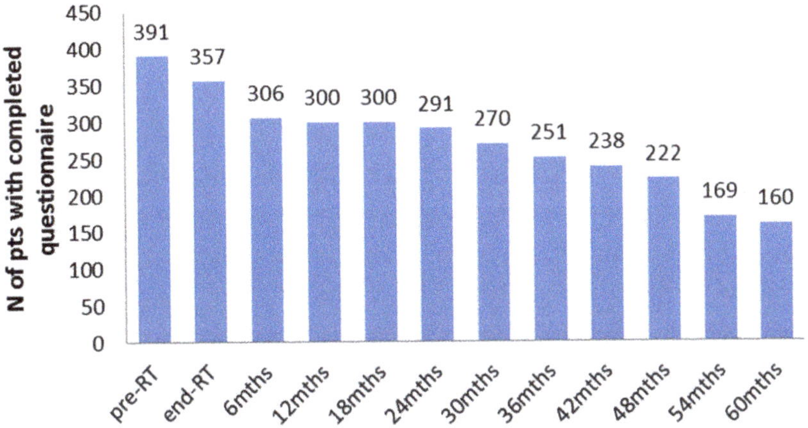

Figure 1. Number of patients that completed the questionnaire at different time points.

The health-related quality of life (HRQoL) of prostate cancer patients was assessed by means of the EORTC QoL 30-item questionnaire (EORTC QLQ-C30) filled in by patients at baseline, at RT end, and thereafter every 6 months up to 5 years after IMRT. The 14 domains investigated by the EORTC QLQ-C30 were the following: global health/QoL, five functional scales (physical, role, cognitive, emotional, and social), and eight symptom scales/items (fatigue, nausea/vomiting, pain, dyspnoea, insomnia, appetite loss, constipation, and diarrhoea). Patients' responses were scored according to the EORTC QLQ-C30 scoring manual [11]. With respect to the functional scores, a higher score indicated better functioning levels, whereas a higher score in the symptom scales indicated a higher severity (worse) of symptoms.

The questionnaire scores were longitudinally evaluated across time using repeated-measures analysis of variance for multiple measures (ANOVA). Effects of multiple variables such as age, presence and type of hormonal therapy, prescribed dose, and CTCAE (Common Toxicity Criteria for Adverse Event, v4.03) acute intestinal Grade $\geq$2 on QoL changes over the time were studied using two-way repeated-measures analysis of variance. Differences among groups were evaluated through the Mann–Whitney test. A p value <0.05 was considered to indicate statistical significance.

The statistical analysis was performed using Medcalc statistical software (Version 10; Broekstratt 52, 9030 Mariakerke, Belgium).

3. Results

3.1. Longitudinal Changes in QoL Scores

The median age of the patients considered was 71 years. Table 3 reports the summary of the results from the ANOVA analysis while Figure 2 presents longitudinal results for the 14 investigated QoL dimensions. A general trend toward the significant worsening of QoL at RT end with respect to the baseline was detected for global health (5-point worsening, $p = 0.05$), physical (4-point worsening, $p = 0.04$), role functioning (5-point worsening, $p = 0.04$), fatigue (7-point worsening, $p = 0.03$), appetite loss (5-point worsening, $p = 0.004$), diarrhoea (14-point worsening, $p = 0.05$), and pain (5-point worsening, $p = 0.03$). With the only exception of physical functioning which exhibited a further worsening of 4 points at 5 years, all the remaining QoL aspects impaired by RT usually recovered within 6 months from radiotherapy conclusion. No significant variations were, on the contrary, observed for cognitive functioning, insomnia, nausea, dyspnoea, and constipation.

Table 3. Results of ANOVA analysis (over 5 years after the end of IMRT) on the 14 QoL dimensions investigated by EORTC QLQ C30 questionnaire.

Qol Dimension	Significant Trend with Time from ANOVA	*p*-Value	Time and Size of Significant Variation
Global health/QoL	quadratic	0.05	5-point worsening at RT end with respect to baseline, then recovery
Physical functioning	cubic	0.04	4-point worsening at RT end with respect to baseline, then recovery, further 4-point worsening at 5 years
Role functioning	cubic	0.04	5-point worsening at RT end with respect to baseline, then recovery, further 5-point worsening at 5 years
Social functioning	linear	0.04	2-point increase in the 5-year period
Emotional functioning	linear	0.01	3-point increase in the 5-year period
Cognitive functioning	no significant trend		
Appetite loss	quadratic	0.004	5-point worsening at RT end with respect to baseline, then recovery
Diarrhoea	quadratic + linear decrease	0.05	14-point worsening at RT end with respect to baseline, then recovery, and at 5 years, 1.5 points better with respect to baseline
Fatigue	quadratic	0.03	7-point worsening at RT end with respect to baseline, then recovery
Insomnia	no significant trend		
Dyspnoea	no significant trend		
Pain	quadratic	0.03	5-point worsening at RT end with respect to baseline, then recovery
Constipation	no significant trend		
Nausea	no significant trend		

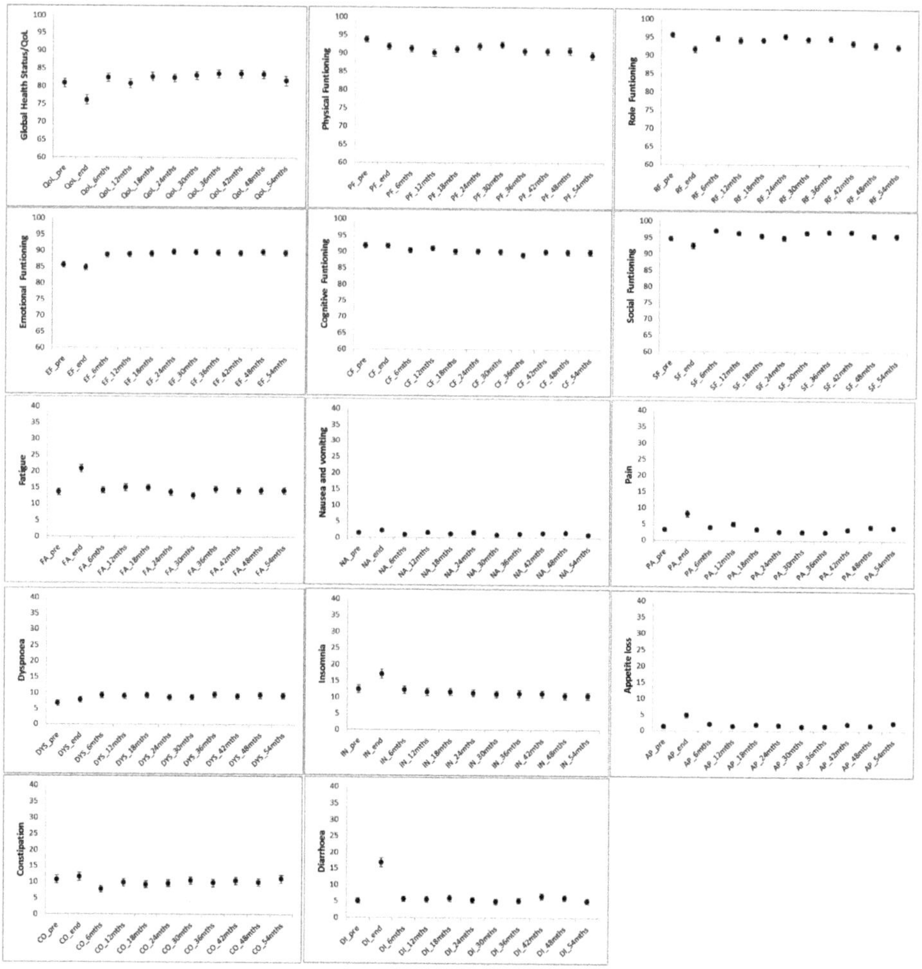

Figure 2. Longitudinal evaluation (5-year time frame of the EORTC QLQ C30 investigated QoL dimensions.

3.2. Predictors of QoL Changes at RT End

Considering the most impaired time point of the ANOVA, detailed analyses focused on the possible predictors' deterioration of HRQoL at RT end were carried out. It emerged that acute Grade $\geq$ 2 GI toxicity significantly impaired global health, physical, role functioning, fatigue, appetite loss, diarrhoea, and pain (p-value range: 0.02–0.0003, worsening range: 3–9 points). Prophylactic lymph-nodal irradiation resulted in significantly lower QoL levels for global health, fatigue, appetite loss, and diarrhoea (p-value range: 0.05–0.0001, worsening range: 5–14 points). Acute Grade $\geq$ 2 GU toxicity led to lower levels of role functioning and higher pain ($p = 0.03$ and 0.002, respectively, worsening 5 and 10 points, respectively). The radiation doses were associated with diarrhoea (most informative cut-off at 81 2Gy-equivalent, $p = 0.0001$, 23.9 vs. 13 points). The use of any neoadjuvant/concomitant hormonal therapy was associated with lower pain (6.7 vs. 11, $p = 0.01$), while the use of a peripheral anti-androgen (e.g., bicalutamide) was associated with lower fatigue (19.2 vs. 24.8, $p = 0.01$).

4. Discussion

Intense research is actively performed not only to improve prostate cancer patient clinical outcomes but also to better understand the possible impact of side effects on an individual's functioning, both physical and psychosocial. These issues may clearly have a strong impact on the patient's decision-making process. In fact, all these items not only reflect the patient's overall physical health but also are related to the ability to perform tasks associated with daily life activities and employment. In this study, we therefore investigated the longitudinal QoL changes from radiotherapy start to 5 years after IMRT-IGRT delivered for PCa within a large multicentric study. The prospective evaluation of HRQoL was performed using patient-reported QoL evaluated by means of a validated questionnaire, the EORTC QLQ-C30. In addition, the possible impact of clinical, technical, and dosimetric data on QoL were investigated, focusing on the timing corresponding to the evidence of a significant impact of the treatment on QoL.

The results of this study highlighted a relatively temporary worsening of 9 QoL dimensions out of 14 at RT end with respect to baseline, with a complete restoration within 6 months, with the sole exception of physical functioning, exhibiting an additional worsening of 4 points at the 5-year follow-up. The disappearance of the detrimental effect in certain aspects of QoL after six months can be explained by the fact that supporting nutritional status, a possible mental health serenity connected to anxiety reduction, suddenly managing symptoms during and following treatment, and good treatment tolerability improve QOL. Moreover, acute symptoms usually resolve within a few months [16] and patients present a fatigue reduction related to the end of transportation to the radiotherapy centre.

In particular, a worsening of 5 points for global health, role functioning, appetite loss, and pain and 4 points for physical functioning were detected at RT end. These findings are consistent with previous reports describing lower HRQoL and functional status following RT [4,11,13,17–19]. On the other hand, some studies reported no significant changes in daily activities during the treatment course [20,21].

The two dimensions mostly impaired by irradiation were fatigue and diarrhoea, which exhibited a worsening of 7 and 14 points, respectively, at radiotherapy end. The more likely sources of fatigue during radiotherapy may be hormonal therapy, transportation to the institute where radiotherapy is delivered, and the treatment itself, while diarrhoea represents the most common radiation side effect related to pelvic radiotherapy. Fatigue is very commonly reported in men treated with radiotherapy for prostate cancer [17,22]. Physical functioning worsening may probably be related to patients' age increasing between baseline and 60 months follow-up. In the series of Sveistrup et al. [23], a decrease in physical functioning one year after RT was observed even though it was usually small (<5 points). The authors' hypothesis was that a decrease in physical functioning lower than 5 points had to be considered clinically not significant. No variation in cognitive functioning, insomnia, nausea, dyspnoea, and constipation was observed in our series. The lack of change in cognitive function following radiotherapy was also reported by Bansal et al. [24]. Other studies showed, on the contrary, moderate but transient impaired QoL immediately after radiotherapy [16,25]. The exact reason for the correlation of a lower degree of pain and hormonal therapy is not easily explainable. A hypothesis could be that the result is influenced by the concept called benefit finding. Namely, benefit finding refers to the fact that the beginning of pharmacological therapy could reduce patient anxiety related to the patient's illness. In fact, it was reported that symptom complications such as fatigue, sleeplessness, pain, and diarrhoea were significantly associated with levels of anxiety [26].

When focusing on QoL dimensions' variation at radiotherapy end as compared to baseline, acute Grade ≥ 2 GI toxicity was found to significantly affect global health, physical, role functioning, fatigue, appetite loss, diarrhoea, and pain, while acute Grade ≥ 2 GU toxicity produced lower role functioning and higher pain. Also, Sveistrup and coworkers [23], analysing the impact of urinary and gastrointestinal bothers, concluded that the worsening of both GU and GI symptoms were associated with a QoL decrease in several scales. Clark et al. [27], investigating the impact of pelvic symptoms on HRQoL scores, reached similar conclusions. Conversely, Jereczek-Fossa et al. [28], considering a cohort of 337 patients followed for 19 months after irradiation, reported no change in urinary symptom-related QoL in PCa patients treated with image-guided radiation therapy.

Prophylactic lymph-nodal irradiation resulted in significantly lower QoL for global health, fatigue, appetite loss, and diarrhoea (p range: 0.05–0.0001, worsening range: 5–14 points), apparently as a result of the larger volumes irradiated. Higher prescription doses were associated with an increased risk of diarrhoea, even though it was only if delivered at radiation doses exceeding 81 EQD2 Gy, possibly as a result of the more refined dose delivery achievable with modern IMRT. The impact of radiation doses on short-term bowel dysfunction, such as diarrhoea, urgency, or rectal pain, is largely reported. Acute symptoms usually resolve within a few months [16].

The use of any neoadjuvant/concomitant hormonal therapy was associated with lower pain (6.7 vs. 11, $p = 0.01$), while the use of an anti-androgen was associated with lower levels of fatigue in the range of 5 points. Sanda et al. [29] highlighted how vitality may be lower in patients who receive androgen deprivation therapy (ADT). Similarly, Langston et al. [22] and Lilleby et al. [17] reported that fatigue is a common side effect in men affected by prostate cancer, especially if receiving ADT. The direct impact of hormonal therapy on fatigue and on treatment-related symptoms was also found by Marchand et al. [30]. It is noteworthy to observe that, differently from what was observed by Krahn MD et al. [18], no impact of ADT on social functioning and global health emerged in our study.

The strength of our series is that all data were collected prospectively, including all the baseline HRQoL data collected prior to the treatment start. Moreover, the 5-year longitudinal nature of study has the potential to adequately capture even slight changes in patients' HRQoL over a robust time span. At the same time, considering the time interval of data collection in the study, it was possible to correlate the changes to specific causes. Similar prior studies mostly reported results at 2 years [31]. Thereafter, our results not only confirm the 6-month prospective published literature data on HRQoL after IMRT [19,32] but also provide additional information of HRQoL trends up to 60 months.

The fact that the patients recovered their initial QoL within 6 months is an extremely important result indicating a good tolerability of the treatment. Therefore, considering that acute toxicity is predictive of late toxicity for general toxicity as well as urinary and bowel toxicity, we will also expect less late toxicity. Moreover, the "acute" effects that disappear after six months could be in favour of hypofractionation that allows for the shortening of the radiotherapy course leading to direct patient convenience, cost savings, and potential radiobiological advantages. In fact, the literature reported that prostate cancer has a relatively low alpha–beta ratio compared to other malignancies, and even in relation to adjacent normal tissues (e.g., rectum and bladder). This suggests an increase in the therapeutic ratio with larger doses per fraction; that is, prostate cancer cells are more sensitive to hypofractionation than the surrounding organs at risk.

In this study, however, we did not have the opportunity to investigate if hormonal therapy for more or less than six months has an impact on QoL and if outcome variation during the patients' follow-up modifies the QoL score.

5. Conclusions

Our findings suggest that modern radiotherapy delivered by conventional or hypofractionated regimens with EQD2 doses up to 90 Gy represents a modality that does not significantly affect long-term QoL. A temporary deterioration of some investigated endpoints was experienced by patients at the end of radiotherapy, but all radiation-induced detrimental effects disappeared after six months from radiotherapy end. This result is extremely important because it indicates that there is no need for additional home health or spousal support.

We believe that nowadays the prostate cancer treatment aim is not only to prolong life, increasing tumour control rate and survival, but also to apply any effort aiming to improve QoL. Moreover, a regular QoL measurement of patients during the treatment course may be a useful instrument in order to detect QoL variation early using a personalized approach.

On the other hand, further analyses should focus on better depicting specific subgroups of patients who may be more subject to long-term impairment of HRQoL.

Author Contributions: Writing—original draft preparation, A.M. (Angelo Maggio), T.R., C.F. and C.C.; data curation, C.B. and F.B.; writing—review and editing, M.G., D.C., B.A., B.F., P.F., T.G., G.G., V.L., A.M. (Alessandro Magli), E.M., E.P., P.S., G.S., E.V., J.M.W., A.G. and R.V. All authors have read and agreed to the published version of the manuscript.

Funding: The research leading to these results has received funding from AIRC under IG 2014-ID. 14603 project—P.I. Cozzarini Cesare.

Institutional Review Board Statement: The study was conducted in accordance with the Declaration of Helsinki, and approved by the Ethics Committee of Fondazione Centro San Raffaele del Monte Tobar Istituto Scientifico Ospedale San Raffaele—Milano (protocol code: DUE-01 and date of approval: 4-3-2010)" for studies involving humans.

Informed Consent Statement: Informed consent was obtained from all subjects involved in the study.

Data Availability Statement: The data presented in this article is not readily available due to privacy and ethical restrictions and because are part of an ongoing study.

Conflicts of Interest: The authors declare no conflict of interest.

References

1. Mottet, N.; Bellmunt, J.; Bolla, M.; Briers, E.; Cumberbatch, M.G.; De Santis, M.; Fossati, N.; Gross, T.; Henry, A.M.; Joniau, S.; et al. EAU-ESTRO-SIOG guidelines on prostate cancer. Part 1: Screening, diagnosis, and local treatment with curative intent. *Eur. Urol.* **2017**, *71*, 618–629. [CrossRef] [PubMed]
2. Wilt, T.J.; MacDonald, R.; Rutks, I.; Shamliyan, T.A.; Taylor, B.C.; Kane, R.L. Systematic review: Comparative effectiveness and harms of treatments for clinically localized prostate cancer. *Ann. Intern. Med.* **2008**, *148*, 435–448. [CrossRef] [PubMed]
3. Chou, R.; Croswell, J.M.; Dana, T.; Bougatsos, C.; Blazina, I.; Fu, R.; Gleitsmann, K.; Koenig, H.C.; Lam, C.; Maltz, A.; et al. Screening for prostate cancer: A review of the evidence for the U.S. Preventive Services Task Force. *Ann. Intern. Med.* **2011**, *155*, 762–771. [CrossRef] [PubMed]
4. Wallis, C.J.; Saskin, R.; Choo, R.; Herschorn, S.; Kodama, R.T.; Satkunasivam, R.; Shah, P.S.; Danjoux, C.; Nam, R.K. Surgery Versus Radiotherapy for Clinically-localized Prostate Cancer: A Systematic Review and Meta-analysis. *Eur. Urol.* **2016**, *70*, 21–30. [CrossRef] [PubMed]
5. Schröder, F.H.; Hugosson, J.; Roobol, M.J.; Tammela, T.L.; Zappa, M.; Nelen, V.; Kwiatkowski, M.; Lujan, M.; Määttänen, L.; Lilja, H.; et al. Screening and prostate cancer mortality: Results of the European Randomised Study of Screening for Prostate Cancer (ERSPC) at 13 years of follow-up. *Lancet* **2014**, *384*, 2027–2035. [CrossRef]
6. Andriole, G.L.; Crawford, E.D.; Grubb, R.L.; Buys, S.S.; Chia, D.; Church, T.R.; Fouad, M.N.; Isaacs, C.; Kvale, P.A.; Reding, D.J.; et al. Prostate cancer screening in the randomized prostate, Lung, Colorectal, and Ovarian Cancer Screening Trial: Mortality results after 13 years of follow-up. *JNCI J. Natl. Cancer Inst.* **2012**, *104*, 125–132. [CrossRef]
7. Chen, R.C.; Rumble, R.B.; Loblaw, D.A.; Finelli, A.; Ehdaie, B.; Cooperberg, M.R.; Morgan, S.C.; Tyldesley, S.; Haluschak, J.J.; Tan, W.; et al. Active surveillance for the management of localized prostate cancer (Cancer Care Ontario guideline): American Society of Clinical Oncology clinical practice guideline endorsement. *J. Clin. Oncol.* **2016**, *34*, 2182–2190. [CrossRef]

8. Donovan, J.L.; Hamdy, F.C.; Lane, J.A.; Mason, M.; Metcalfe, C.; Walsh, E.; Blazeby, J.M.; Peters, T.J.; Holding, P.; Bonnington, S.; et al. Patient-reported outcomes after monitoring, surgery, or radiotherapy for prostate cancer. *N. Engl. J. Med.* **2016**, *375*, 1425–1437. [CrossRef]
9. Sureda, A.; Fumadó, L.; Ferrer, M.; Garín, O.; Bonet, X.; Castells, M.; Mir, M.C.; Abascal, J.M.; Vigués, F.; Cecchini, L.; et al. Health-related quality of life in men with prostate cancer undergoing active surveillance versus radical prostatectomy, external-beam radiotherapy, prostate brachytherapy and reference population: A cross-sectional study. *Health Qual. Life Outcomes* **2019**, *17*, 11. [CrossRef] [PubMed]
10. Yucel, B.; Akkaş, E.A.; Okur, Y.; Eren, A.A.; Eren, M.F.; Karapınar, H.; Babacan, N.A.; Kılıçkap, S. The impact of radiotherapy on quality of life for cancer patients: A longitudinal study. *Support. Care Cancer* **2014**, *22*, 2479–2487. [CrossRef] [PubMed]
11. Fayers, P.M.; Aaronson, N.K.; Bjordal, K.; Groenvold, M.; Curran, D.; Bottomley, A.; on behalf of the EORTC Quality of Life Group. *The EORTC QLQ-C30 Scoring Manual*, 3rd ed.; European Organisation for Research and Treatment of Cancer: Brussels, Belgium, 2001.
12. Carillo, V.; Cozzarini, C.; Rancati, T.; Avuzzi, B.; Botti, A.; Borca, V.C.; Cattari, G.; Civardi, F.; Degli Esposti, C.; Franco, P.; et al. Relationships between bladder dose–volume/surface histograms and acute urinary toxicity after radiotherapy for prostate cancer. *Radiother. Oncol.* **2014**, *111*, 100–105. [CrossRef]
13. Cozzarini, C.; Rancati, T.; Carillo, V.; Civardi, F.; Garibaldi, E.; Franco, P.; Avuzzi, B.; Degli Esposti, C.; Girelli, G.; Iotti, C.; et al. Multi-variable models predicting specific patient-reported acute urinary symptoms after radiotherapy for prostate cancer: Results of a cohort study. *Radiother. Oncol.* **2015**, *116*, 185–191. [CrossRef]
14. Fowler, J.A. The radiobiology of prostate cancer including new aspects of fractionated radiotherapy. *Acta Oncol.* **2005**, *44*, 265–276. [CrossRef] [PubMed]
15. Fiorino, C.; Cozzarini, C.; Rancati, T.; Briganti, A.; Cattaneo, G.M.; Mangili, P.; Di Muzio, N.G.; Calandrino, R. Modelling the impact of fractionation on late urinary toxicity after postprostatectomy radiation therapy. *Int. J. Radiat. Oncol. Biol. Phys.* **2014**, *90*, 1250–1257. [CrossRef] [PubMed]
16. Zelefsky, M.J.; Poon, B.Y.; Eastham, J.; Vickers, A.; Pei, X.; Scardino, P.T. Longitudinal assessment of quality of life after surgery, conformal brachytherapy, and intensity-modulated radiation therapy for prostate cancer. *Radiother Oncol.* **2016**, *118*, 85–91. [CrossRef] [PubMed]
17. Lilleby, W.; Stensvold, A.; Dahl, A.A. Fatigue and other adverse effects in men treated by pelvic radiation and long-term androgen deprivation for locally advanced prostate cancer. *Acta Oncol.* **2016**, *55*, 807–813. [CrossRef] [PubMed]
18. Krahn, M.D.; E Bremner, K.; Tomlinson, G.; Naglie, G. Utility and health-related quality of life in prostate cancer patients 12 months after radical prostatectomy or radiation therapy. *Prostate Cancer Prostatic Dis.* **2009**, *12*, 361–368. [CrossRef] [PubMed]
19. Namiki, S.; Ishidoya, S.; Tochigi, T.; Kawamura, S.; Kuwahara, M.; Terai, A.; Yoshimura, K.; Numata, I.; Satoh, M.; Saito, S.; et al. Health-related quality of life after intensity modulated radiation therapy for localized prostate cancer: Comparison with conventional and conformal radiotherapy. *Ultrasound Med. Biol.* **2006**, *36*, 224–230. [CrossRef] [PubMed]
20. Monga, U.; Kerrigan, A.J.; Thornby, J.; Monga, T.N.; Zimmermann, K.P. Longitudinal study of quality of life in patients with localized prostate cancer undergoing radiotherapy. *J. Rehabil. Res. Dev.* **2005**, *42*, 391–400. [CrossRef]
21. Caffo, O.; Amichetti, M.; Mussari, S.; Romano, M.; Maluta, S.; Tomio, L.; Galligioni, E. Physical side-effects and quality of life during postoperative radiotherapy for uterine cancer. Prospective evaluation by a diary card. *Gynecol. Oncol.* **2003**, *88*, 270–276. [CrossRef]
22. Langston, B.; Armes, J.; Levy, A.; Tidey, E.; Ream, E. The prevalence and severity of fatigue in men with prostate cancer: A systematic review of the literature. *Support. Care Cancer* **2013**, *21*, 1761–1771. [CrossRef]
23. Sveistrup, J.; Mortensen, O.S.; Bjørner, J.B.; Engelholm, S.A.; Rosenschöld, P.M.A.; Petersen, P.M. Prospective assessment of the quality of life before, during and after image guided intensity modulated radiotherapy for prostate cancer. *Radiat. Oncol.* **2016**, *11*, 117. [CrossRef]
24. Bansal, M.; Mohanti, B.; Shah, N.; Chaudhry, R.; Bahadur, S.; Shukla, N. Radiation related morbidities and their impact on quality of life in head and neck cancer patients receiving radical radiotherapy. *Qual. Life Res.* **2004**, *13*, 481–488. [CrossRef] [PubMed]
25. Lips, I.M.; van Gils, C.H.; van der Heide, U.A.; Kruger, A.E.B.; van Vulpen, M. Health-related quality of life 3 years after high-dose intensity-modulated radiotherapy with gold fiducial marker-based position verification. *BJU Int.* **2009**, *103*, 762–767. [CrossRef] [PubMed]
26. Gogou, P.; Tsilika, E.; Parpa, E.; Kouvaris, I.; Damigos, D.; Balafouta, M.; Mystakidou, V.M.A.K. The Impact of Radiotherapy on Symptoms, Anxiety and QoL in Patients with Cancer. *Anticancer. Res.* **2015**, *35*, 1771–1776. [PubMed]
27. Clark, J.A.; Rieker, P.; Propert, K.J.; A Talcott, J. Changes in quality of life following treatment for early prostate cancer. *Urology* **1999**, *53*, 161–168. [CrossRef] [PubMed]
28. Jereczek-Fossa, B.A.; Santoro, L.; Zerini, D.; Fodor, C.; Vischioni, B.; Dispinzieri, M.; Bossi-Zanetti, I.; Gherardi, F.; Bonora, M.; Caputo, M.; et al. Image guided hypofractionated radiotherapy and quality of life for localized prostate cancer: Prospective longitudinal study in 337 patients. *J. Urol.* **2013**, *189*, 2099–2103. [CrossRef]
29. Sanda, M.G.; Dunn, R.L.; Michalski, J.; Sandler, H.M.; Northouse, L.; Hembroff, L.; Lin, X.; Greenfield, T.K.; Litwin, M.S.; Saigal, C.S.; et al. Quality of life and satisfaction with outcome among prostate-cancer survivors. *N. Engl. J. Med.* **2008**, *358*, 1250–1261. [CrossRef] [PubMed]

30. Marchand, V.; Bourdin, S.; Charbonnel, C.; Rio, E.; Munos, C.; Campion, L.; Bonnaud-Antignac, A.; Lisbona, A.; Mahé, M.-A.; Supiot, S. No impairment of quality of life 18 months after high-dose intensity-modulated radiotherapy for localized prostate cancer: A prospective study. *Int. J. Radiat. Oncol. Biol. Phys.* **2010**, *77*, 1053–1059. [CrossRef] [PubMed]
31. Alemozaffar, M.; Regan, M.M.; Cooperberg, M.R.; Wei, J.T.; Michalski, J.M.; Sandler, H.M.; Hembroff, L.; Sadetsky, N.; Saigal, C.S.; Litwin, M.S.; et al. Prediction of erectile function following treatment for prostate cancer. *JAMA* **2011**, *306*, 1205–1214. [CrossRef]
32. Lips, I.; Dehnad, H.; Kruger, A.B.; van Moorselaar, J.; van der Heide, U.; Battermann, J.; van Vulpen, M. Health-related quality of life in patients with locally advanced prostate cancer after 76 gy intensity-modulated radiotherapy vs. 70 gy conformal radiotherapy in a prospective and longitudinal study. *Int. J. Radiat. Oncol. Biol. Phys.* **2007**, *69*, 656–661. [CrossRef] [PubMed]

Current Oncology

MDPI

Systematic Review

From CBCT to MR-Linac in Image-Guided Prostate Cancer Radiotherapy Towards Treatment Personalization

Florentina Larisa Coc [1,2] and Loredana G. Marcu [3,4,*]

1 Faculty of Physics, West University of Timisoara, 300223 Timisoara, Romania; larisa.coc@e-uvt.ro
2 Bihor County Emergency Clinical Hospital, 410167 Oradea, Romania
3 Faculty of Informatics & Science, University of Oradea, 410087 Oradea, Romania
4 Allied Health & Human Performance, University of South Australia, Adelaide, SA 5001, Australia
* Correspondence: loredana@marcunet.com

Abstract: Purpose: Image-guided radiotherapy (IGRT) has been widely implemented in the treatment of prostate cancer, offering a number of advantages regarding the precision of dose delivery. This study provides an overview of factors, clinical and physical alike, that increase treatment accuracy in prostate cancer radiotherapy in the context of IGRT. The following aspects are explored based on recent literature: the radiotherapy technique used in conjunction with IGRT, the type and frequency of IGRT, the impact of radiotherapy technique/IGRT on target dosimetry and organs at risk, the influence of IGRT on planning target volume margins, the impact of treatment time on dosimetric outcome and clinical outcomes using IGRT repositioning or an online adaptive plan. **Methods**: A systematic search of the literature was conducted within Pubmed/Medline databases to find relevant studies. Of the 152 articles fulfilling the initial search criteria, 79 were selected for final analysis. **Results**: The frequency of image guidance, the treatment regimen and the radiation technique are important factors that contribute to the optimization and personalization of the treatment plan. The daily anatomy and volume of the bladder and rectum can vary considerably, which can significantly impact the dosimetric effects on these organs. When used in conjunction with volumetric modulated arc therapy, IGRT allows for shaping the dose distribution to avoid nearby critical structures such as the bladder and rectum. **Conclusions**: Precise tumor targeting via IGRT can result in fewer geometric uncertainties, thereby improving treatment outcome both in terms of superior target coverage and sparing organs at risk.

Keywords: image-guided radiotherapy; geometric errors; PTV margin; organs at risk; adaptive radiotherapy; tumor control; quality of life

1. Introduction

According to the latest statistics, prostate cancer (PCa) is the second most common cancer in men in Western Europe and the United States and the fourth most common cancer overall [1]. External beam radiotherapy (EBRT) is the main treatment option for many patients diagnosed with PCa owing to increased efficiency compared to other treatment techniques [2]. In recent years, radiotherapy has undergone significant advancements, enabling the delivery of a more precise and conformal dose to the prostate while simultaneously reducing the dose to surrounding organs at risk (OARs) [3]. In view of this, three-dimensional conformal radiation therapy (3D CRT) has been replaced by techniques employing intensity-modulated beams, such as IMRT (intensity-modulated radiotherapy) or VMAT (volumetric modulated arc therapy) [4]. Yet, compared to 3D CRT, IMRT has some acknowledged disadvantages, such as increased monitor units (MUs) and longer treatment delivery time (even double), which can result in higher positioning errors [5]. For instance, if the treatment time were to be doubled from 1 to 2 min, software analysis suggests that the prostate may move between 750 and 1500 times over the treatment course [6]. VMAT was shown to overcome these drawbacks through the use of arcs or semi-arcs to deliver the treatment in a continuous rotation of the gantry [5].

Both IMRT and VMAT require high accuracy in tumor localization due to possible variations in patient positioning caused by setup errors. Image-guided radiotherapy (IGRT) techniques, when used in conjunction with IMRT or VMAT, can significantly improve treatment accuracy. IGRT techniques include two-dimensional megavoltage (MV) or kilovoltage (kV) imaging, cone-beam computed tomography (CBCT) and megavoltage computed tomography (MVCT). Additionally, non-radiative techniques, such as ultrasound, the Calypso system, the AlignRT system or magnetic resonance imaging (MRI), can be employed to monitor the position of the prostate in real time. One of the key roles of IGRT in prostate cancer radiotherapy is to increase treatment precision and to reduce the planning target volume (PTV) margins for better conformity and organ sparing [2].

While radiotherapy delivery aims for high precision, there are factors that can limit accuracy. It is important to note that errors can occur despite all efforts to minimize them. These errors are the result of a number of factors, such as tumor motion, weight loss, and changes in patient posture or organ volumes. In addition to interfractional variations, it is essential to consider intrafractional variations caused by internal physiological movements such as breathing, rectal gas, swallowing or heartbeat. To ensure accurate treatment, it is necessary to (re)optimize the treatment plan with appropriate PTV margins, taking into account the movement of the prostate. Differences in PTV margins may occur due to variations in the frequency of IGRT techniques, time intervals between IGRT and treatment, and differences in bladder and rectal filling from one radiotherapy session to the next [7].

Adaptive radiotherapy (ART) is a solution that adjusts treatment plans according to these changes. ART can be conducted in two ways: online, with adjustments made during treatment sessions, or offline, with adjustments made between sessions [8]. The MR-Linac has numerous advantages, including improved anatomic visualization of OARs, being a potential treatment approach for reirradiation of prostate cancer after intraprostatic recurrence while also offering the option for direct soft-tissue-based gating [9]. However, MR images are prone to geometric distortions when treating patients with metal prostheses/implants [10], and treatment time may be prolonged (up to 45–60 min) [11].

The purpose of this study is to provide an overview of factors contributing to treatment precision and personalization in prostate cancer radiotherapy in the context of IGRT. To fulfil this aim, the following aspects were investigated based on the published literature: EBRT used in combination with IGRT; the IGRT method and frequency; the impact of technique/IGRT on target and OAR dosimetry, including reoptimization or adaptive radiotherapy; the decision on PTV margins according to IGRT indications; and the effect of treatment time on dosimetric and clinical outcomes.

2. Methods—Literature Search

This systematic review is reported according to the 2020 PRISMA (Preferred Reporting Items for Systematic Review and Meta-Analysis) guidelines, and it has been registered with the Open Science Framework with the registration code OSF.IO/342MR being available at: https://osf.io/rmavj (accessed on 12 April 2025).

The search of the literature was conducted within the Pubmed/Medline databases for scientific articles published over the past 10 years (2014–2025) using the following as keywords: "prostate cancer" AND "intensity modulated radiotherapy OR IMRT OR volumetric modulated radiotherapy OR VMAT" AND "image-guided radiation therapy OR IGRT". Studies were included regardless of tumor stage or treatment status, as long as the patients received external radiotherapy. The present study exclusively considers full-text articles that focus on male patients and are written in English. Reviews, abstracts and conference proceedings were excluded. As a result, 493 articles met the search criteria. The search was narrowed down to articles focusing on treatment personalization using the keywords "PTV margins" and "adaptive radiotherapy". Article filtration was thus facilitated, resulting in the identification of 152 publications (74 pertaining to PTV margins and 78 to adaptive radiotherapy). Articles concerning fewer than 10 patients or non-EBRT (brachytherapy), as well as articles that provide only radiation effects on hematological parameters or those not presenting a quantitative dose analysis, were excluded, leading to 79 eligible articles (Figure 1).

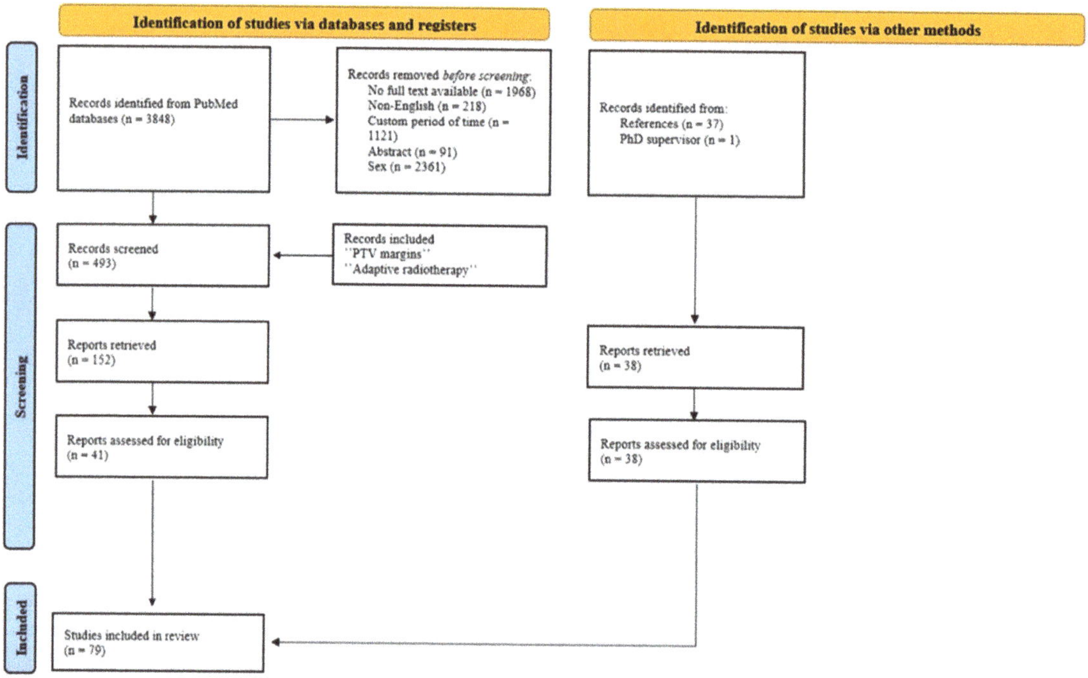

Figure 1. PRISMA flow diagram for literature search.

3. Results

3.1. Imaging Techniques Used on Board the Linear Accelerator to Guide Prostate Cancer Treatment

To increase treatment precision delivery, modern treatment techniques have incorporated pretreatment imaging to account for, prevent and/or correct any patient or organ movement that may occur. Several IGRT techniques are implemented in clinics, and the most common ones, together with their prevalence in prostate cancer radiotherapy, are shown in Figure 2.

Based on the last 10 years' statistics, **CBCT** is the most commonly employed imaging method in prostate radiotherapy, with 41% of the analyzed articles reporting its regular use. CBCT provides better visualization of the bladder and rectum, though at the expense of higher imaging dose, particularly for MV systems (EPID MV 30–70 mGy/image, EPID kV 1–3 mGy/image, CBCT 30–50 mGy/image), and a twofold acquisition time [12].

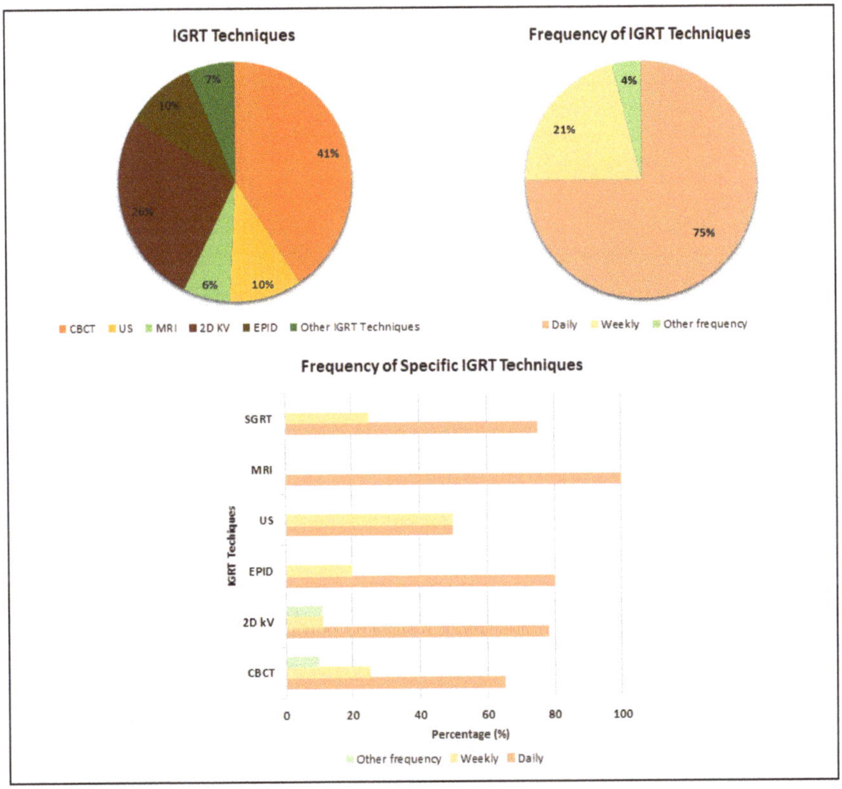

Figure 2. Most commonly used IGRT techniques and their frequency in prostate cancer radiotherapy.

As shown in Figure 2, another commonly used IGRT method applied in 26% of cases reported in the literature is two-dimensional **orthogonal kV imaging with or without fiducial markers** (FM). FM can facilitate the tracking of inter- or intrafractional movements of the prostate; therefore, FM-based IGRT is an effective tool that can increase the accuracy of radiotherapy while minimizing the radiation dose to normal tissues [13].

Magnetic resonance imaging (MRI) has been integrated into linear accelerators to create MR-Linac systems (MRIgRT) to facilitate adaptive treatments and motion management. The primary advantage of this technology is the superior soft-tissue contrast it provides [14], as well as its capacity to control intrafraction motion without the need for additional dose to the patient [15].

Surface-Guided Radiotherapy (SGRT) creates 3D images of the patient's surface, which are compared to a reference surface to assist with positioning. Using SGRT for prostate cancer provided a faster and more accurate patient positioning compared to the conventional three-point localization setup [16].

Ultrasound imaging offers an alternative solution for verifying the treatment setting in order to quantify changes in bladder and rectal filling levels, as it is a non-invasive and non-radiative procedure [17].

Figure 2 illustrates **the frequency of IGRT** use in prostate cancer radiotherapy as conveyed from the literature. While most centers reported daily usage of IGRT, around 20% employ image guidance for prostate radiotherapy on a weekly basis. A limited number of clinics reported other IGRT regimens, including the use of IGRT for the first 3 days of treatment, followed by weekly imaging every other day or daily for the first week, followed by once-a-week imaging. The technique, which is used less frequently on a daily basis, is either in the initial stages of implementation or is employed in conjunction with other IGRT techniques.

A limited number of studies evaluated the association between the type/frequency of image guidance and treatment-related adverse effects [18,19]. In their IMRT study, Serizawa et al. compared the outcomes and toxicities of patients treated with IGRT using fiducial markers vs. patients treated without image guidance (non-IGRT). The IGRT cohort was divided into the IGRT-A group, which used the same margins as the non-IGRT group, and the IGRT-B group, with reduced margins. In comparison with non-IGRT, the IGRT-A group showed a lower rate of grade 2+ late GU toxicities (16% vs. 28%), as well as a lower rate of grade 1+ acute GI toxicities (44% vs. 55%). Furthermore, when compared to the IGRT-A group, the IGRT-B group had reduced rates of acute grade 2+ GU (21% vs. 45%) and acute grade 1+ GI toxicities (18% vs. 44%), illustrating the protective role of reduced tumor margins on the adjacent organs at risk [18].

Ghanem et al. compared the impact of daily (arm A) vs. irregular IGRT (arm B), with arm A undergoing IMRT with daily CBCT and arm B patients being positioned on skin tattoos, with 3D-US or 2D KV scans performed on a weekly or biweekly basis. Arm A presented fewer grade 2 (18.1% vs. 28.6%) and grade 3 (1.4% vs. 6.5%) late GU toxicities than arm B, with the most common late GU toxicities being irritative symptoms, hematuria and urethral stricture [19]. The study reiterated the role of frequent (daily) IGRT for accurate targeting, which, inherently, leads to better normal tissue protection.

3.2. *Positioning Errors in Prostate Cancer Treatment*

A patient setup error is defined as a discrepancy between the actual and expected position of the patient relative to the treatment beam, recorded along the X, Y and Z axes, respectively. These errors are then corrected according to each department's protocol [20]. Setup errors can extend to a six-degree (6D) scope (three translational and three rotational setup errors). Unfortunately, rotational setup errors are not routinely corrected because most currently available couches can only correct one degree of these rotational movements [21]. Motion variation within a fraction is referred to as intrafractional error, while the variation between fractions is designated as interfractional error. These errors have been classified into random (σ) and systematic (Σ), and for each setting, they are calculated based on inter- and intrafractional changes in the prostate. Random errors are statistical fluctuations (alterations in the patient's position and internal anatomy, such as those resulting from respiration, bladder filling, or rectal distention), while systematic ones are often due to a problem that persists throughout the treatment (difficulties in target delineation due to tumor regression or growth, discrepancies in laser alignment between CT and linear accelerator, or isocenter location) [22,23]. Their timely identification and implementation of counteracting measures are essential [23,24].

Based on the above-mentioned setup verification systems, Table S1 presents positioning errors as reported by the literature in terms of interfractional and intrafractional errors.

3.2.1. Interfractional Error Management in Prostate IGRT

The minimization of interfractional errors can be achieved through the implementation of optimal IGRT, facilitating real-time imaging of the prostate. Alternatively, an increase in the frequency of IGRT can be used to reduce the incidence of inaccuracies.

To evaluate the advantages and limitations of various IGRT techniques, Mayyas et al. performed a comparative study employing three different IGRT modalities: 3D ultrasound, kV planar imaging and CBCT (Figure 3). The correlation between the shifts evaluated by CBCT and 2D kV was found to be high in the LR and AP directions but low in the SI direction. This may be related to the difficulty in accurately visualizing the prostate apex and base on CBCT. A lower correlation was also observed between 2D kV and US in the AP direction. The time interval between scans (CBCT followed by 2D kV and US, with a minimum of a 10 min delay between the CBCT and US) is a potential explanation for the observed differences, as setup and physiological changes could have occurred between the initial CBCT and the US scan. The interfractional errors were the highest for US (mean error in AP direction −1.2 mm CBCT; −2.9 mm 2D kV; −3.6 mm US). This study also provides insight into the additional dose due to imaging scans throughout treatment: five CBCT scans per week at 2 cGy/scan or five orthogonal image pairs/week at 0.1 cGy/image added approximately 98 cGy additional dose to the treatment [25].

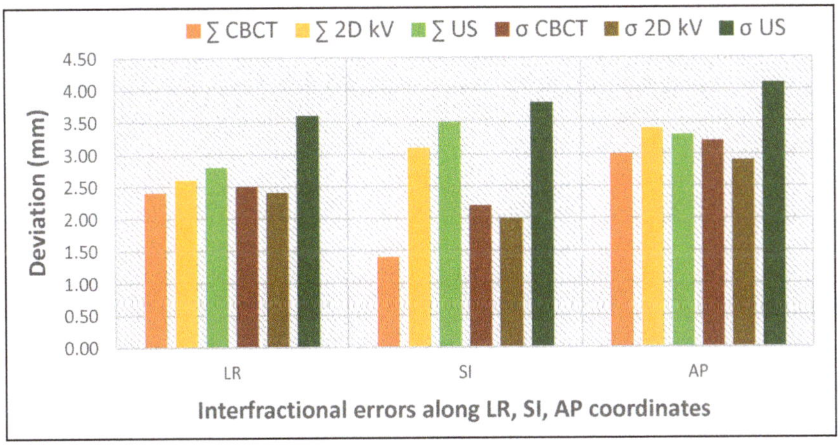

Figure 3. Impact of different IGRT techniques on interfractional errors (based on data from [25]).

Krengli et al. compared the daily variations detected by two non-ionizing IGRT techniques, 3D surface imaging and transabdominal ultrasound, to examine the configuration of prostate and internal organ variation (Figure 4). Systematic errors detected by 3D surface and 3D US imaging were significantly different only in the LR direction, which was caused by the difficulty in precisely defining the lateral border of the prostate by ultrasound. Therefore, these two techniques could be used as complementary quality assurance methods and could serve as a daily non-invasive IGRT technique in prostate radiotherapy [26].

Rosenschöld et al. highlighted the importance of IGRT frequency while comparing alternative pretreatment image guidance protocols by using the first fraction weekly and daily. The study demonstrated that weekly 2D kV compared to the initial treatment session resulted in a reduction in systematic errors (from 0.15, 0.26, 0.21 to 0.08, 0.12, 0.09 (mm)), but the random errors remained high (from 0.28, 0.42, 0.29 to 0.35, 0.29, 0.37 (mm) on the lateral, longitudinal and vertical axes, respectively). Additionally, it was observed that in patients with an elevated body mass index, a more rigorous IGRT protocol is necessary, such as daily IGRT. The implementation of regular IGRT in this patient group reduced random errors to 0.1 mm on all three axes [27].

Liu et al. analyzed interfractional organ motion after prostatectomy, evaluating three treatment plans for the same patient: a plan using IGRT repositioning, an online adaptive plan by adapting the original plan to conform to the anatomy of the day and a new plan reoptimized entirely based on the daily anatomy. Data from the study showed that online replanning can correct both systematic and random errors and has the advantage of keeping the original dose distribution throughout the treatment sessions [28].

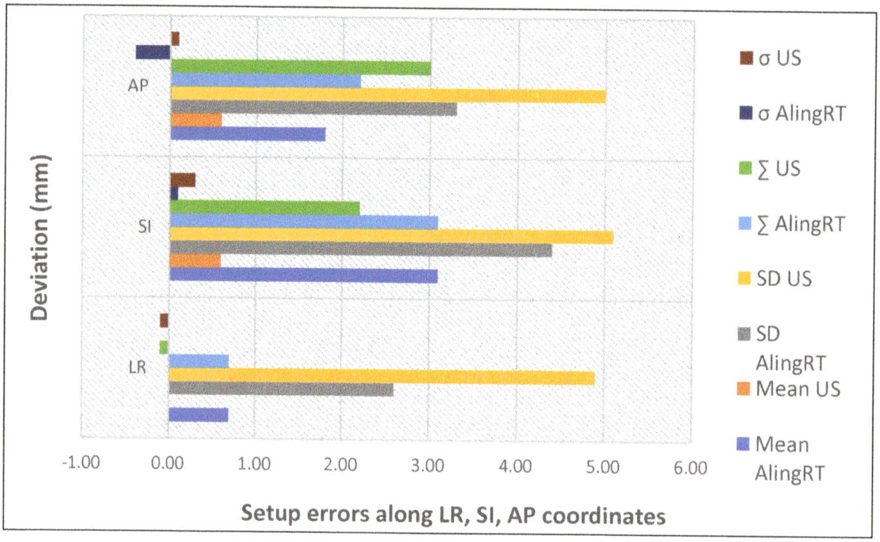

Figure 4. Setup errors quantified by non-invasive IGRT (based on data from [26]).

Figure 5 illustrates the mean setup errors for the main IGRT techniques used in prostate cancer, as analyzed by this review [13,25,26,29–39]. The mean error is generally used to denote the systematic setup error, which is defined as the average deviation between the planned and actual patient positions across all treatment fractions. The data reveal that CBCT improves positioning precision due to the 3D reference. Planar kV images are quick but only show bony structures, whereas CBCT highlights soft tissues, offering a higher positioning accuracy. Also, while the data show that US imaging can offer similar accuracy to CBCT in pretreatment positioning, generally, it is not safely interchangeable with the latter due to poorer image quality. Recent advancements in MR-Linac technology have significantly increased its use for assessing prostate intrafraction motion. This rise is due to improved soft tissue contrast, continuous imaging without added dose, and the elimination of the need for fiducial markers.

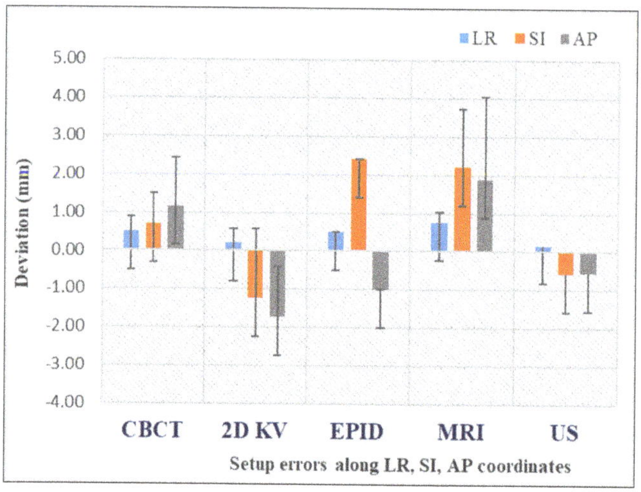

Figure 5. Mean setup errors for various IGRT techniques. The bars represent the standard deviation of the dataset relative to the mean.

3.2.2. Intrafractional Error Management in Prostate IGRT

Intrafractional movement of the prostate is assessed by considering changes in target position relative to bony anatomy, tracking based on fiducial markers or electromagnetic transponders. From the analysis of the literature and data quantification in Table S1, it can be concluded that intrafractional movement of the prostate is influenced by the degree of bladder filling, rectal diameter and the size and shape of the prostate.

The study conducted by Ballhausen et al. demonstrated that the length of treatment is a significant factor influencing the extent of intrafractional movement of the prostate. The intrafractional motion of the prostate was recorded by real-time four-dimensional ultrasound (4DUS) in 28 patients, 14 being treated with step-and-shoot IMRT, while the other 14 patients were treated with VMAT. The mean prostate radial displacement per fraction was found to be substantially and significantly reduced, from 1.31 $\pm$ 1.28 mm (n = 357 IMRT fractions) to 0.96 $\pm$ 1.04 mm (n = 363 VMAT fractions). The prostate remained at 4.55 mm distance from the isocenter for 95% of the fraction time during IMRT and at 2.45 mm distance during VMAT. The variance of the displacements increased linearly with time [40].

For optimal treatment delivery, Tatar et al. recommend MR-guided radiotherapy with daily plan adaptation. They observed that prostate coverage was achieved in 49 out of 50 fractions with a 5 mm PTV without plan adaptation. However, coverage of the seminal vesicles (SVs) was insufficient in 15 out of 50 fractions, which was corrected through adaptive radiotherapy while reducing intrafractional motion [41].

3.3. *The Influence of Positioning Errors on the PTV Margin*

A personalized treatment plan in prostate cancer radiotherapy can only be created with appropriate PTV margins; thus, there are several recommended methods for calculating these margins (see, for example, [42]):

- ICRU Report 62: PTV margin = $\sum + 0.7\sigma$,
- Stroom's method: PTV margin = $2\sum + 0.7\sigma$,
- Van Herk's formula: PTV margin = $2.5\sum + 0.7\sigma$.

In addition to the size of errors, several factors can affect the PTV margin, such as CTV margins, tumor cell density, tumor cell aggressiveness and heterogeneity, as well as the vicinity of normal structures [23]. The PTV margins reported by prostate studies published in the literature are shown in Table S2. In most studies, the PTV margins were calculated based on pretreatment CBCT images using the Van Herk formula.

For example, Su et al. showed that fiducial marker matching results in the smallest PTV margins for the prostate (1.5 + 0.2 mm, 3.5 + 0.5 mm, 2.7 + 0.4 mm in LR, SI and AP direction, respectively), while bone matching leads to the smallest PTV margins for the lymph nodes (0.7 + 0.1 mm, 1.5 + 0.2 mm, 1.4 + 0.2 mm in LR, SI and AP direction, respectively). On the other hand, tattoo matching led to the highest PTV margins, approximately double compared to matching on FM, for both prostate and lymph nodes, the latter being increased due to the interfractional movement of the prostate relative to the pelvic bones [43]. Within the same context, Mayyas et al. reported that each technique (US, kV and CBCT) provided additional information on the reproducibility of the prostate configuration during treatment and reduced the PTV margin by 4 mm compared to alignment on tattoos [25].

Furthermore, Ghaffari et al. reported a set of PTV margins in their daily EPID study (4.0 mm, 3.3 mm and 3.0 mm in the lateral, longitudinal and vertical axes, respectively), which, in the absence of daily verification and correction, would be required to increase (5.4 mm, 5.8 mm and 5.5 mm along the LR, SI and AP directions, respectively) to achieve a 95% CTV coverage [44].

Recent studies indicate that the most effective reduction in PTV margin while maintaining the prescribed dose to the prostate is achieved via MR-Linac due to real-time adjustments in target geometry and volume during adaptive radiotherapy: 65% of patients moved less than 2 mm in any direction during movement monitoring period, while 30% moved 3 mm [45,46].

Figure 6 illustrates the differences between the PTV margin established in the planning phase and the PTV margin calculated using the van Herk formula, after accounting for systematic and random errors using IGRT [20,29,38,47–52]. This graph underscores the significance of IGRT in prostate radiotherapy, demonstrating the way monitoring prostate movement enables the optimization of treatment plans by reducing the margin while maintaining the accuracy of dose delivery to the CTV and minimizing exposure to critical structures. The largest discrepancies between the planning and calculated PTV margins occurred along the LR direction. In contrast, PTV margins along the SI and AP directions resulted in smaller discrepancies. It is plausible that the observed change in the AP and SI directions was due to patient relaxation or a change in bladder and rectal fullness. This also demonstrates the necessity of an anisotropic edge. Treatment margins should be patient-dependent or individualized to maximize the benefit of conformal dose distributions in VMAT and IMRT.

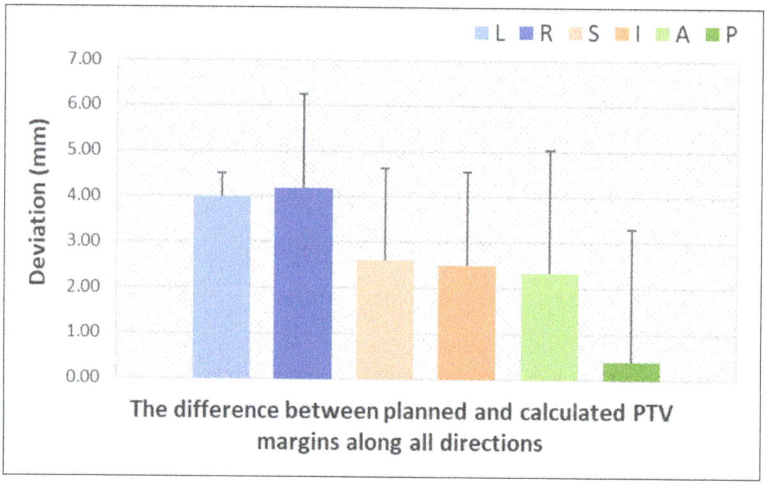

Figure 6. Quantification of setup errors by IGRT techniques (based on data from Table S2) (L = left; R = right; S = superior; I = inferior; A = anterior; P = posterior). The bars represent the standard deviation of the dataset relative to the mean.

3.4. Dosimetric Impact of PTV Margin Optimization on Target Coverage and OARs

The impact of geometric errors and PTV margins on dose distribution, hot and cold spots and tumor volume coverage in prostate cancer radiotherapy are summarized in Supplementary Table S3.

Table S4 summarizes the dosimetric values estimated for the rectum and bladder as the main organs at risk, based on the published literature. Dosimetric parameters for the femoral head and other organs less frequently reported in the literature (such as the sigmoid colon, the penile bulb and the urethra) are also shown in this table.

In the study reported by Li et al., the impact of PTV margin on dosimetric parameters pertaining to the rectum and urinary bladder was observed, as well as the difference between planned and delivered dose. It seems that there is a correlation between the reduction in PTV margins and the decreased exposure of healthy tissue to radiation.

This is evidenced by the decrease in the D25 parameter with PTV margin reduction for both the rectum and bladder, which dropped from 52.8% to 41.95% and from 54.07% to 47.70%, respectively. Upon recalculation of the dose distributions on the CBCT images, it became evident that there were notable variations, particularly in the rectum, where D50 increased from 39.20% to 41.11%. Similarly, in the case of the bladder, its fullness appeared to contribute to the observed change, with the dose decreasing from 32.7% to 31.48%. These observations confirm the potential benefit of daily IGRT in prostate cancer radiotherapy [53].

The objective of the study conducted by Heng et al. was to ascertain the impact of bladder and bowel preparation protocols on dosimetric outcome using IMRT planning and CBCT evaluation of the above organs. A total of 12 patients were included in the study, with 6 undergoing the bladder and bowel preparation protocol and the other 6 serving as the control group. The contoured volumes of the bladder and rectum on CBCT images were compared with those on the planning CT. All patients were treated with a total dose of 78 Gy in 39 fractions over a period of 8 weeks. A comparison of patients with and without a bladder preparation protocol revealed that patients without such instructions presented with a greater bladder volume and a higher degree of dose variation. The maximum variation in rectal volume on the day of treatment was found to be up to +96% due to changes in rectal filling. In contrast, the maximum variations in rectal volume with the bowel preparation protocol were less than 25%. The data confirmed that a rectum and bladder preparation protocol can improve treatment accuracy while also leading to reduced side effects and enhanced quality of life [54].

Plan Adaptation and Its Impact on Setup Errors

Given that IGRT is unable to fully account for patient-specific treatment variations, the strategy of plan adaptation was introduced with the objective of reducing systematic and random errors. Consequently, Böckelmann et al. devised a clinical approach to evaluate setup errors during treatment sessions for each patient. The initial fractions were employed to assess patient positioning by comparing the planning CT with CBCT scans. In the event of a high degree of concordance between CT and CBCT images, indicating minimal displacement of the rectal balloon and anterior rectal wall, PCa patients were not subjected to an adapted treatment plan. When setup errors indicated greater uncertainties (i.e., the rectal balloon and anterior rectal wall were situated outside the delineated rectal volume), a new planning CT scan was conducted, an adapted set of contours was created, and a treatment plan was developed that adhered to the principles of adapted interfractional patient positioning accuracy for both the initial and adapted treatment plans. The displacements in the LR and SI directions were smaller for the adapted plan (1.12 and 1.72 mm for Σ and 4.17 and 3.75 mm for σ) than for the original plan (1.77 and 2.62 mm for Σ and 4.46 and 5.39 mm for σ). With regard to AP motion, the adapted (1.73 mm for Σ and 3.20 for σ) and initial (1.67 mm for Σ and 3.21 for σ) plans were observed to exhibit comparable characteristics. The CTV-PTV margin in the AP direction demonstrated comparable outcomes, with a range of 6–8 mm between the original and adapted plans. Conversely, the LR and SI margins of the adapted plans showed reductions of 2 mm (5–6 mm and 7–8 mm) and 3 mm (7–8 mm and 10–11 mm), respectively, in comparison to the margins derived from the original plans [47].

Mannerberg et al. investigated the role of adaptive radiotherapy in 35 PCa patients based on two MR images (MR1 and MR2) taken 30 min apart using an MR-Linac. Three ultra-hypofractionated VMAT plans were created based on MR1 with three different PTV margins (7 mm, 5 mm and 3 mm), the plans being recalculated using the second set of MR images (MR2). Results showed an increase in bladder volume by an average of 40.9%

between the two images. The difference in rectal volume ranged from 10.9% to 38.8%, with the negative differences in rectal volume being caused by gas. The dose to the CTV was reduced by 1.1% with the 7 mm PTV margin. The corresponding values for 5 mm and 3 mm PTV margins were 2.0% and 4.2%, respectively. While the results confirm the role of adaptive treatment in personalized radiotherapy, the authors suggest that, owing to the slow MR-Linac workflow, target underdosage can occur due to anatomical changes during the investigation [16].

3.5. *The Impact of Treatment Time on Error Reduction*

Shorter treatment times in radiotherapy are directly associated with a reduction in intrafractional motion and delivery uncertainties. For instance, a study by Li et al. has shown that hypofractionated VMAT treatment is effective in reducing treatment time, as compared to IMRT. VMAT delivers the dose in 2–4 min, while conventional IMRT treatment takes 3–7 min. Owing to this, a 7 mm isotropic margin (5 mm posterior) was used in the conventional group, while a 5 mm isotropic margin (4 mm posterior) was used in the hypofractionated group. When dose distributions were recalculated using CBCT images, the results showed that VMAT plans offer better PTV D95% and a reduction in most dosimetric parameters pertaining to organs at risk [53]. In addition, Benedeka et al. showed that using VMAT without a flattening filter for the ultra-hypofractionated delivery of radiation reduces treatment time by around 50% (from 2.3 min to 1.01 min), while keeping the dosimetric effect of organ movement under control. There was no deterioration in the quality of the treatment plan in terms of dose volume parameters or delivery plan verification results [24].

In terms of treatment duration and its impact on plan quality, VMAT was found to demonstrate superiority over three other techniques (3D CRT, 5-field IMRT, helical tomotherapy (HT)). VMAT was better at reducing rectal and bladder toxicity and allowed for a higher dose to the target. The highest MUs were obtained with the HT technique, leading to an average treatment delivery time of 4.70 ± 0.84 min as compared to 3D CRT (0.74 ± 0.04 min), IMRT (1.42 ± 0.26 min) and VMAT (0.87 ± 0.06 min) [55].

The technology and design of the latest linear accelerators allow for further optimization of treatment delivery. In view of this, Pokhrel et al. evaluated the performance of the O-ring Halcyon in prostate cancer in terms of quality, delivery efficiency and accuracy. Two types of stereotactic body radiotherapy (SBRT) plans were generated: one with a Halcyon beam of 6MV-FFF (800 MU/min) and the other with a TrueBeam beam of 6MV-FFF (1400 MU/min). Despite the longer beam start times for Halcyon plans (3.2 min, up to 3.8 min) in comparison to TrueBeam VMAT plans (2.1 min, up to 2.5 min), the total treatment times are comparable, with a mean delivery time of 8.20 ± 0.46 min for the Halcyon linac and 9.90 ± 0.19 min for the traditional C-arm linac [56].

4. Discussion

The potential of IGRT to enhance the effectiveness of radiotherapy treatment for patients diagnosed with prostate cancer is well understood, provided that the technology is efficiently utilized. In this context, several studies present the advantages and limitations of IGRT techniques.

For instance, an advantage of CBCT consists of the overlay of 3D reference data with the pretreatment acquisition. This is performed either manually or automatically following one of three procedures: bone alignment, soft tissue alignment (ST) or dual alignment. Some studies have shown that the PTV margins based on soft tissue alignment are smaller than those based on bony structure [29,48]. This translates into a lower risk of late rectal toxicity [57]. However, a study reported by Hirose et al. showed the efficiency of 2D-FM parameters in defining PTV margins, as compared to CBCT-ST, to reduce the risk of under-irradiation [49]. Although fiducial markers can be used to indicate the position of the prostate, they are not capable of conveying the shape of the prostate in real time.

Modern radiotherapy centers are in a position to benefit from the high resolution of MRI. Consequently, prostate cancer studies using MRIgRT have reported an isotropic PTV margin reduction to 3 mm, in contrast with 5 mm with CT-guided RT [58]. Other radiotherapy centers have adopted alternative IGRT techniques (such as SGRT or US), which have been shown to be more cost-effective and better suited to meet the specific resources of each department. Some limitations of the SGRT technique include the presence of hair on the patient's skin surface, which can compromise the accuracy of positioning due to the loss of surface calculation points [59]. Additionally, daily variations in bladder and bowel filling, which are not evident on the patient's surface, can also introduce challenges. Also, a number of studies have demonstrated that configurations based on user-dependent transperineal ultrasound (TPUS) and user-independent CBCT lead to large geometric differences, especially in the anteroposterior (AP) direction [30,31]. In light of these discrepancies, it was concluded that ultrasound fails to provide an acceptable level of geometric accuracy for prostate localization. Consequently, these techniques are recommended to be employed in conjunction with other IGRT techniques [60]. This could provide a non-invasive, daily option for prostate cancer patients [26].

The use of IGRT and its frequency can influence decisions regarding the reduction of the PTV margin to achieve better OAR protection while still maintaining the prescribed dose within the volume of interest. For instance, Ariyaratne et al. showed that 90% of patients achieved better target coverage with daily compared to weekly CBCT imaging [61].

Advancements in technology have facilitated more precise monitoring of tumor variations. Initially, tattoo positioning was utilized; subsequently, bony marking was employed; and, finally, fiducial markers were introduced for the identification of soft tissues. In the current era, 3D pretreatment information can be obtained, and even real-time tracking of prostate variations is now possible. Consequently, positioning errors in prostate cancer treatment have been significantly minimized. A number of studies demonstrate the advantage of using fiducial markers for position verification, showing smaller systematic errors in seed matching than in bony matching on the lateral and vertical axes [13,43,49,50]. They also confirmed that random errors associated with seed matching are more significant than those associated with bony matching on the same axes. This may be caused by the motion of the pelvic lymph node, which is influenced by bladder filling and small intestine motion [43].

On the other hand, the advantages of high-quality soft tissue contrast for MR-Linac have shown that bone registration, with or without FM, cannot be a perfect surrogate for prostate registration; therefore, online adaptive planning is required for accurate treatment delivery. Nikol et al. used three FMs and observed that the FMs migrated by 0.05 mm/fraction due to prostatic deformation [62], while Kim et al. observed interfractional variability based on bone anatomy and prostate registration, showing a strong correlation only in the AP direction: mean error 0.57, 2.28, 2.45 (mm) after bone localization and 0.76, 2.02, 1.89 (mm) after prostate localization on the lateral and vertical axes [32]. This finding aligns with numerous others that have hypothesized that MR-Linac and online adaptive radiotherapy could facilitate the reduction of prostate motion during treatment, and PTV margins could be safely reduced to 3 mm [41,63,64].

It can be seen from the evidence presented above that each IGRT technique has its own particular advantages and drawbacks. It is thought that the most accurate solution in patient positioning includes a daily MRI, although many centers use a CBCT/2D kV system with fiducial markers. However, if the patient is not eligible for the insertion of fiducial markers, it may be beneficial to consider combining CBCT or 2D kV with non-ionizing IGRT ultrasonography or 3D surface imaging, allowing movement monitoring in real time.

Studies to date suggest that it is difficult, if not impossible, to completely eliminate all geometric errors during prostate radiotherapy. However, daily IGRT was shown to significantly reduce PTV margins [51].

It is to be noted that successfully achieving optimal dosimetry for one criterion, e.g., PTV coverage, is often in conflict with meeting the requirements for the other criterion, i.e., the restrictions imposed by OARs. There are situations when complications are acceptable; in the case of volumetrically applied dose constraints, this means that the risk of complications depends on the dose distributed throughout the organ. In contrast, for serial organs, complications due to geometric errors are unacceptable, and the risk of complications depends strongly on the region receiving the maximum dose [65].

As most studies indicate, the quality of target volume coverage increases as the PTV margin increases. However, increasing the PTV margin has the downside of high toxicity to organs at risk. Therefore, it is necessary to explore other methods to maintain clinically adequate tumor volume coverage while keeping the PTV margin low. For this purpose, many radiotherapy clinics follow a prostate cancer protocol in which the patient is scanned with a full bladder and empty rectum [54]. The movement of the prostate is limited by these two organs at risk to ensure that the tumor volume receives the planned radiation dose.

Despite advances in treatment planning and delivery, the rectum remains a critical organ that raises caution in prostate cancer patients undergoing radiotherapy. Radiation-induced rectal toxicities continue to be a clinical challenge due to the close proximity of the anterior rectal wall to the prostate gland. Physical devices such as endorectal balloons, hydrogel rectal spacers or rectal retractors have been used to increase the distance between the prostate and the rectum [43]. In addition to these devices, IGRT has allowed for a reduction of the PTV margin in the posterior region [66]. The use of anisotropic margins was shown to increase the probability of tumor control while decreasing normal tissue effects.

Da Silva et al. argued that the determination of the PTV margins depends on the pretreatment imaging system used. In their study, comparable plan quality was obtained between CBCT-guided VMAT plans and MRI-guided IMRT plans using the same PTV margin [1]. However, MRI-guided online adaptive radiotherapy allowed for margin reduction, owing to the additional soft tissue information provided by this imaging technique.

Although MRI is superior to CBCT in terms of OAR dosimetry [14], when compared to 2D pretreatment techniques, CBCT remains advantageous in certain instances. Nakamura et al. found that IMRT with soft tissue-matched CBCT allows for a reduction of the PTV margin without compromising tumor control, which successfully reduced acute rectal toxicity compared to IMRT configured on 2D bone landmarks [2]. Furthermore, Maund et al. suggested that the use of IMRT in conjunction with daily CBCT could result in a reduction of the PTV margin from 5 mm to 3 mm without compromising tumor control and is favorable in terms of reducing rectal toxicity. At the same time, they cautioned that a smaller margin presents a challenge due to the interfractional movement of seminal vesicles [67]. These findings highlight the importance of frequent imaging in achieving better treatment accuracy and increased therapeutic index in radiotherapy [31].

Thus, in order to minimize the discrepancy between the planned and delivered doses, it is essential to ensure that the patient follows the protocol for filling the urinary bladder and emptying the rectum, thereby achieving a volume as close as possible to that on the day of the CT simulation. Rectal and urinary bladder variations can be compensated for by an additional margin. However, this approach also has a disadvantage reflected by the increased radiation-induced toxicity, which can often be tackled by adaptive radiotherapy.

This review has identified numerous studies evaluating the accuracy of dose delivery using different IGRT in prostate cancer. A comparison between reports is challenging due to the large number of variables identified among the evaluated studies, such as image acquisition protocol, frequency of IGRT, treatment planning system (TPS) algorithm and the diversity of dosimetric parameters reported in the articles. However, it seems that previous studies have indicated that MR-Linac represents a future-oriented solution for adaptive radiotherapy in prostate cancer.

As for current challenges, the implementation of online adaptive radiotherapy requires considerable investment in capital, equipment and personnel, which represents a substantial barrier to its adoption. For instance, the Elekta Accelerator has developed a new mechanism that enables position adaptation (online plan adaptation is performed based on the new patient's position and optimized on the pretreatment CT and contours) and shape adaptation (online plan adaptation is performed on the new patient's anatomy and optimized on the daily MRI and adapted contours). This allows for the visualization of all anatomical changes during the course of radiotherapy, enabling the adaptation of the treatment plan to ensure optimal results [68].

Another critical aspect of online adaptive MRgRT is that it is time-consuming, not only because MRI is inherently slow, but also due to the multi-step adaptation process. The online adaptation can extend the radiotherapy sessions by 30 to 60 min, impacting treatment efficacy [69]. In this context, the use of high-resolution IGRT that allows for automatic alignment, combined with a hypofractionated treatment regimen, was shown to be among the optimal solutions for delivering effective and rapid treatment [16].

A promising direction for adaptive MRgRT involves the use of quantitative MRI-derived biomarkers, which can provide valuable information about treatment response, allowing clinicians to detect tumor microenvironmental changes that could indicate early responses or resistance to treatment [70]. Current trends show that online adaptive MRI-guided radiotherapy is transforming conventional treatment workflows while also integrating advanced AI-assisted processes to boost efficiency and maintain high standards of dosimetric accuracy during treatment delivery [71].

5. Conclusions

Image-guided radiotherapy techniques are key tools in enhancing tumor control by identifying and correcting positioning errors in real time. The type of such technology, frequency of use, and the PTV margins, as well as the target position relative to organs at risk, are all critical factors that dictate treatment outcome. Intensity-modulated treatment techniques were shown to offer a more precise and targeted approach to the tumor, minimizing toxicity and providing superior protection of normal tissues compared to conventional techniques. Furthermore, patients' compliance regarding prostate cancer treatment protocols (bladder/rectal filling) has an important impact on internal organ movement and should be strictly monitored on a daily basis during the course of radiotherapy. This, in turn, has the potential to enhance the patient's quality of life.

The role of CBCT in the precise delivery of prostate cancer radiotherapy has been proven by several studies, being considered a key component of the treatment process and an important factor leading to a more personalized treatment approach. It is evident that MRI offers a number of advantages; however, this technology remains accessible to a limited number of centers due to the significant financial investment required. Therefore, most centers use CBCT in conjunction with other IGRT systems (e.g., ultrasound or surface-guided radiotherapy) to increase the precision of prostate cancer radiotherapy.

A summary of the main findings based on the analyzed literature is collated below:

- CBCT is the most frequently employed IGRT technique, representing 41% of pretreatment imaging in prostate cancer radiotherapy.
- Daily IGRT verification improves target volume coverage in 90% of patients compared with weekly imaging.
- To avoid the risk of underdosing the tumor volume, the PTV margin must be kept at 3 mm or above, especially in situations when IGRT is not used daily.
- When patient positioning is based on skin tattoo vs. IGRT, it is recommended for the PTV margin to be doubled.
- As confirmed by a number of studies, VMAT has the advantage of reducing the intrafractional displacement variation of the prostate by half when compared to IMRT.
- Among linac-based techniques, VMAT provides optimal-quality treatment plans, offering a reduction of up to 50% in monitor units and treatment time while achieving the most conformal isodoses.
- MRI-guided radiotherapy represents the next solution for individualized and adaptive treatment in prostate cancer patients.

Supplementary Materials: The following supporting information can be downloaded at: https://www.mdpi.com/article/10.3390/curroncol32060291/s1, Table S1. Types of interfractional and intrafractional errors and their identification by IGRT in prostate radiotherapy (studies are listed in chronological order) [13,20,22,25–27,29–39,43,44,47–52,72–79]; Table S2. PTV margin reduction in prostate cancer treatment according to the literature [20,22,25,29,32,33,35,37–39,43,44,47–52,72,78–80] Table S3. PTV-related dosimetric parameters based on the literature (studies are listed in chronological order) [1,5,16,28,51–53,55,56,61,64,66,77,80–92]; Table S4. Dosimetric parameters evaluated for the OARs during prostate cancer radiotherapy (studies are listed in chronological order) [2,4,5,16,28,34, 41,53,55,56,61,64,66,77,80–91,93–97].

Author Contributions: All authors contributed to the study conception and design. Data collection and analysis were performed by F.L.C., original draft was written by F.L.C. and L.G.M., and review and editing were performed by F.L.C. and L.G.M. All authors have read and agreed to the published version of the manuscript.

Funding: This research received no external funding.

Conflicts of Interest: The authors declare no conflicts of interest.

References

1. Mendes, V.D.S.; Nierer, L.; Li, M.; Corradini, S.; Reiner, M.; Kamp, F.; Niyazi, M.; Kurz, C.; Landry, G.; Belka, C. Dosimetric comparison of MR-linac-based IMRT and conventional VMAT treatment plans for prostate cancer. *Radiat. Oncol.* **2021**, *16*, 133. [CrossRef] [PubMed]
2. Nakamura, K.; Mizowaki, T.; Inokuchi, H.; Ikeda, I.; Inoue, T.; Kamba, T.; Ogawa, O.; Hiraoka, M. Decreased acute toxicities of intensity-modulated radiation therapy for localized prostate cancer with prostate-based versus bone-based image guidance. *Int. J. Clin. Oncol.* **2017**, *23*, 158–164. [CrossRef]
3. Fischer-Valuck, B.V.; Rao, Y.J.; Michalski, J.M. Intensity-modulated radiotherapy for prostate cancer. *Transl. Androl. Urol.* **2018**, *7*, 297–307. [CrossRef] [PubMed]
4. Zhao, H.; Sarkar, V.; Wang, B.; Rassiah-Szegedi, P.; Szegedi, M.; Huang, Y.J.; Huang, L.; Tward, J.; Salter, B. Calculation of delivered composite dose from Calypso tracking data for prostate cancer: And subsequent evaluation of reasonable treatment interruption tolerance limits. *J. Appl. Clin. Med. Phys.* **2019**, *20*, 105–113. [CrossRef]
5. Kinhikar, R.A.; Pawar, A.B.; Mahantshetty, U.; Murthy, V.; Dheshpande, D.D.; Shrivastava, K.S. Rapid Arc, helical tomotherapy, sliding window intensity modulated radiotherapy and three dimensional conformal radiation for localized prostate cancer: A dosimetric comparison. *J. Cancer Res. Ther.* **2021**, *10*, 575–582. [CrossRef] [PubMed]
6. Varnava, M.; Sumida, I.; Oda, M.; Kurosu, K.; Isohashi, F.; Seo, Y.; Otani, K.; Ogawa, K. Dosimetric comparison between volumetric modulated arc therapy planning techniques for prostate cancer in the presence of intrafractional organ deformation. *J. Rad. Res.* **2021**, *62*, 309–318. [CrossRef]

7. Emin, S. Feasibility of Adaptive SBRT of Prostate Cancer: Investigating Uncertainties in AI-Driven and CBCT-Guided Online Adaptive Radiotherapy. Master's Thesis, Lund University, Lund, Sweden, 2020.
8. Lemus, O.M.D.; Cao, M.; Cai, B.; Cummings, M.; Zheng, D. Adaptive Radiotherapy: Next-Generation Radiotherapy. *Cancers* **2024**, *16*, 1206. [CrossRef]
9. Benitez, C.M.; Steinberg, M.L.; Cao, M.; Qi, S.; Lamb, M.J.; Kishan, A.U.; Valle, F.L. MRI-Guided Radiation Therapy for Prostate Cancer: The Next Frontier in Ultrahypofractionation. *Cancers* **2023**, *15*, 4657. [CrossRef]
10. Keesman, R.; Van der Bijl, E.; Janssen, T.M.; Vijlbrief, T.; Pos, F.J.; Van der Heide, U.A. Clinical Workflow for Treating Patients with a Metallic Hip Prosthesis Using Magnetic Resonance Imaging-Guided Radiotherapy. *Phys. Imaging Radiat. Oncol.* **2020**, *15*, 85–90. [CrossRef]
11. Güngör, G.; Serbez, I.; Temur, B.; Gür, G.; Kayalılar, N.; Mustafayev, T.Z.; Korkmaz, L.; Aydın, G.; Yapıcı, B.; Atalar, B.; et al. Time Analysis of Online Adaptive Magnetic Resonance–Guided Radiation Therapy Workflow According to Anatomical Sites. *Pract. Radiat. Oncol.* **2020**, *11*, e11–e21. [CrossRef]
12. Goyal, S.; Kataria, T. Image Guidance in Radiation Therapy: Techniques and Applications. *Radiol. Res. Pract.* **2014**, *2014*, 705604. [CrossRef] [PubMed]
13. Goff, P.H.; Harrison, L.B.; Furhang, E.; Ng, E.; Bhatia, S.; Trichter, F.; Ennis, R.D. 2D Kv orthogonal imaging with fiducial markers is more precise for daily image guided alignments than soft-tissue cone beam computed tomography for prostate radiation therapy. *Adv. Radiat. Oncol.* **2017**, *2*, 420–428. [CrossRef] [PubMed]
14. Kishan, A.U.; Ma, T.M.; Lamb, J.M.; Casado, M.; Wilhalme, H.; Low, D.A.; Sheng, K.; Sharma, S.; Nickols, N.G.; Pham, J.; et al. Magnetic Resonance Imaging-Guided vs Computed Tomography-Guided Stereotactic Body Radiotherapy for Prostate Cancer: The MIRAGE Randomized Clinical Trial. *JAMA Oncol.* **2023**, *9*, 365–373. [CrossRef]
15. Boldrini, L.; Romano, A.; Chiloiro, G.; Corradini, S.; De Luca, V.; Verusio, V.; D'Aviero, A.; Castelluccia, A.; Alitto, A.R.; Catucci, F.; et al. Magnetic Resonance Guided SBRT Reirradiation in Locally Recurrent Prostate Cancer: A Multicentric Retrospective Analysis. *Radiat. Oncol.* **2023**, *18*, 84. [CrossRef] [PubMed]
16. Mannerberg, A.; Kügele, M.; Hamid, S.; Edvardsson, S.; Petersson, K.; Gunnlaugsson, A.; Back, S.A.J.; Engelholm, S.; Ceberg, S. Faster and more accurate patient positioning with surface guided radiotherapy for ultra-hypofractionated prostate cancer patients. *Tech. Innov. Patient Support Radiat. Oncol.* **2021**, *19*, 41–45. [CrossRef]
17. Camps, S.M.; Fontanarosa, D.; Verhaegen, F.; Vanneste, B.G.L. The Use of Ultrasound Imaging in the External Beam Radiotherapy Workflow of Prostate Cancer Patients. *BioMed Res. Int.* **2018**, *2018*, 7569590. [CrossRef]
18. Serizawa, I.; Kozuka, T.; Soyano, T.; Sasamura, K.; Kamima, T.; Kunogi, H.; Kurihara, N.; Numao, N.; Yamamoto, S.; Yonese, J.; et al. Clinical and Dosimetric Comparison Between Non-image Guided Radiation Therapy and Fiducial-Based Image Guided Radiation Therapy With or Without Reduced Margin in Intensity Modulated Radiation Therapy for Prostate Cancer. *Adv. Radiat. Oncol.* **2024**, *9*, 101612. [CrossRef]
19. Ghanem, A.I.; Elsaid, A.A.; Elshaikh, M.A.; Khedr, G.A. Volumetric-Modulated Arc Radiotherapy with Daily Image-Guidance Carries Better Toxicity Profile for Higher Risk Prostate Cancer. *Asian Pac. J. Cancer Prev.* **2021**, *22*, 61–68. [CrossRef]
20. Kanakavelu, N.; Samue, J.J. Determination of patient set-up error and optimal treatment margin for intensity modulated radiotherapy using image guidance system. *Off. J. Balk. Union. Oncol.* **2016**, *21*, 505–511.
21. Amro, H.; Hamstra, D.; Mcshan, D.; Sandler, H.; Vineberg, K.; Hadley, S. The Dosimetric Impact of Prostate Rotations During Electromagnetically Guided External Beam Radiation Therapy. *Int. J. Rad. Oncol. Biol. Phys.* **2014**, *85*, 230–236. [CrossRef]
22. Oehler, C.; Lang, S.; Dimmerling, P.; Bolesch, C.; Kloeck, S.; Tini, A.; Glanzmann, C.; Najafi, Y.; Studer, G.; Zwahlen, D.R. PTV margin definition in hypofractionated IGRT of localized prostate cancer using cone beam CT and orthogonal image pairs with fiducial markers. *Radiat. Oncol.* **2014**, *9*, 229. [CrossRef] [PubMed]
23. Van Herk, M. Errors and Margins in Radiotherapy. *Semin. Rad. Oncol.* **2014**, *14*, 52–64. [CrossRef]
24. Benedeka, H.; Lernera, M.; Nilssona, P.; Knöösa, T.; Gunnlaugssona, A.; Cebergb, C. The effect of prostate motion during hypofractionated radiotherapy can be reduced by using flattening filter free beams. *Phys. Imaging Radiat. Oncol.* **2018**, *6*, 66–70. [CrossRef]
25. Mayyas, E.; Chetty, I.J.; Chetvertkov, M.; Wen, N.; Neicu, T.; Nurushev, T.; Ren, L.; Lu, M.; Stricker, H.; Pradhan, D.; et al. Evaluation of multiple image-based modalities for image-guided radiation therapy (IGRT) of prostate carcinoma: A prospective study. *Med. Phys.* **2013**, *40*, 041707. [CrossRef]
26. Krengli, M.; Loi, G.; Pisani, C.; Beldì, D.; Apicella, G.; Amisano, V.; Brambilla, M. Three dimensional surface and ultrasound imaging for daily IGRT of prostate cancer. *Radiat. Oncol.* **2016**, *11*, 159. [CrossRef] [PubMed]
27. af Rosenschöld, P.M.; Desai, N.B.; Oh, J.H.; Apte, A.; Hunt, M.; Kalikstein, A.; Mechalakos, J.; Happersett, L.; Deasy, J.O.; Zelefsky, M.J. Modeling positioning uncertainties of prostate cancer external beam radiation therapy using pre-treatment data. *Radiother. Oncol.* **2014**, *110*, 251–255. [CrossRef] [PubMed]
28. Liu, F.; Ahunbay, E.; Lawton, C.; Li, X.L. Assessment and management of interfractional variations in daily diagnostic-quality-CT guided prostate-bed irradiation after prostatectomy. *Med. Phys.* **2014**, *41*, 031710. [CrossRef]

29. Sato, H.; Abe, E.; Utsunomiya, S.; Kaidu, M.; Yamana, N.; Tanaka, K.; Ohta, A.; Obinata, M.; Liu, J.; Kawaguchi, G.; et al. Superiority of a soft tissue-based setup using cone-beam computed tomography over a bony structurebased setup in intensity-modulated radiotherapy for prostate cancer. *J. Appl. Clin. Med. Phys.* **2015**, *16*, 239–245. [CrossRef]
30. Richter, A.; Polat, B.; Lawrenz, I.; Weick, S.; Sauer, O.; Flentje, M.; Mantel, F. Initial results for patient setup verification using transperineal ultrasound and cone beam CT in external beam radiation therapy of prostate cancer. *Radiat. Oncol.* **2016**, *11*, 147. [CrossRef]
31. Fargier-Voiron, M.; Presles, B.; Pommier, P.; Munoz, A.; Rit, S.; Sarrut, D.; Biston, M.-C. Ultrasound versus Cone-beam CT image-guided radiotherapy for prostate and post-prostatectomy pretreatment localization. *Phys. Medica* **2015**, *31*, 997–1004. [CrossRef]
32. Kim, J.; Sung, J.; Lee, J.S. Optimal planning target margin for prostate radiotherapy based on interfractional and intrafractional variability assessment during 1.5T MRI-guided radiotherapy. *Front. Oncol.* **2023**, *13*, 1337626. [CrossRef] [PubMed]
33. Adamczyk, M.; Piotrowski, T.; Adamiak, E.; Malicki, J. Dosimetric consequences of prostate-based couch shifts on the precision of dose delivery during simultaneous IMRT irradiation of the prostate, seminal vesicles and pelvic lymph nodes. *Phys. Med.* **2014**, *30*, 228–233. [CrossRef]
34. Hirose, Y.; Nakamura, M.; Tomita, T.; Kitsuda, K.; Notogawa, T.; Miki, K.; Nakamura, K.; Ishigaki, T. Evaluation of different set-up error corrections on dose–volume metrics in prostate IMRT using CBCT images. *J. Radiat. Res.* **2014**, *55*, 966–975. [CrossRef]
35. Shiraishi, K.; Futaguchi, M.; Haga, A.; Sakumi, A.; Sasaki, K.; Yamamoto, K.; Igaki, H.; Ohtomo, K.; Yoda, K.; Nakagawa, K. Validation of planning target volume margins by analyzing intrafractional localization errors for 14 prostate cancer patients based on three-dimensional cross-correlation between the prostate images of planning CT and intrafraction cone-beam CT during volumetric modulated arc therapy. *BioMed Res. Int.* **2014**, *2014*, 960928.
36. Rastogi, M.; Nanda, S.S.; Gandhi, A.K.; Dalela, D.; Khurana, R.; Mishra, S.P.; Srivastava, A.; Farzana, S.; Bhatt, M.L.B.; Husain, N. Pelvic bone anatomy vs implanted gold seed marker registration for image-guided intensity modulated radiotherapy for prostate carcinoma: Comparative analysis of inter-fraction motion and toxicities. *J. Egypt. Nat. Cancer Inst.* **2017**, *29*, 185–190. [CrossRef]
37. Wang, G.; Wang, W.L.; Liu, Y.Q.; Dong, H.M.; Hu, Y.X. Positioning error and expanding margins of planning target volume with kilovoltage cone beam computed tomography for prostate cancer radiotherapy. *OncoTargets Ther.* **2018**, *11*, 1981–1988. [CrossRef] [PubMed]
38. Ingrosso, G.; Miceli, R.; Ponti, E.; Lancia, A.; di Cristino, D.; de Pasquale, F.; Bove, P.; Santoni, R. Interfraction prostate displacement during image-guided radiotherapy using intraprostatic fiducial markers and a cone-beam computed tomography system: A volumetric off-line analysis in relation to the variations of rectal and bladder volumes. *J. Cancer Res. Ther.* **2019**, *15*, 69–75. [CrossRef] [PubMed]
39. Oh, Y.; Baek, J.; Kim, O.; Kim, J. Assessment of setup uncertainties for various tumor sites when using daily CBCT for more than 2200 VMAT treatments. *J. Appl. Clin. Med. Phys.* **2020**, *15*, 85–99. [CrossRef]
40. Ballhausen, H.; Li, M.; Ganswindt, U.; Belka, C. Shorter treatment times reduce the impact of intra-fractional motion. *Strahlenther. Onkol.* **2019**, *194*, 664–674. [CrossRef]
41. Tetar, S.U.; Bruynzeel, A.M.E.; Verweij, L. Magnetic resonance imaging-guided radiotherapy for intermediate- and high-risk prostate cancer: Trade-off between planning target volume margin and online plan adaption. *Phys. Imaging Radiat. Oncol.* **2022**, *23*, 92–96. [CrossRef]
42. Mandal, A.; Singh, P.; Bera, S.; Kumar, A.; Singh, D.; Verma, M.; Rakesh, A.; Sinha, A. Set-up Errors and Determination of Planning Target Volume Margins Protocol for Different Anatomical Sites in a Newly Established Tertiary Radiotherapy Centre in India. *Asian J. Oncol.* **2020**, *6*, 81–87. [CrossRef]
43. Su, Z.; Li, Z.; Henderson, R.; Hoppe, B.S.; Nichols, R.C.; Bryant, C.; Mendenhall, W.; Mendenhall, N. PTV Margin Analysis for Prostate Patients Treated with Initial Pelvic Nodal IMRT and Prostate Proton Boost. *Phys. Med. Biol.* **2019**, *64*, 04NT04. [CrossRef] [PubMed]
44. Ghaffari, H.; Navaser, M.; Mofid, B.; Mahdavi, S.R.; Mohammadi, R.; Tavakol, A. Fiducial markers in prostate cancer image-guided radiotherapy. *Med. J. Islam. Repub. Iran.* **2019**, *33*, 15. [CrossRef] [PubMed]
45. Wahlstedt, I.; Andratschke, N.; Behrens, C.P. Gating has a negligible impact on dose delivered in MRI-guided online adaptive radiotherapy of prostate cancer. *Radiother. Oncol.* **2022**, *170*, 205–212. [CrossRef]
46. de Muinck Keizer, D.M.; de Groot-van Breugel, E.N.; Raaymakers, B.W.; Lagendijk, J.J.; de Boer, H.C. On-line daily plan optimization combined with a virtual couch shift procedure to address intrafraction motion in prostate magnetic resonance guided radiotherapy. *Phys. Imaging Radiat. Oncol.* **2021**, *19*, 90–95. [CrossRef]
47. Böckelmann, F.; Putz, F.; Kallis, K.; Lettmaier, S.; Fietkau, R.; Bert, C. Adaptive radiotherapy and the dosimetric impact of inter- and intrafractional motion on the planning target volume for prostate cancer patients. *Strahlenther. Onkol.* **2020**, *196*, 647–656. [CrossRef]

48. Iwama, K.; Yamazaki, H.; Nishimura, T.; Oota, Y.; Aibe, H.; Nakamura, S.; Ikeno, H.; Yoshida, K.; Okabe, H. Analysis of Intrafractional Organ Motion for Patients with Prostate Cancer Using Soft Tissue Matching Image-guided Intensity-modulated Radiation Therapy by Helical Tomotherapy. *Anticancer. Res.* **2014**, *33*, 5675–5680.
49. Hirose, K.; Sato, M.; Hatayama, Y.; Kawaguchi, H.; Komai, F.; Sohma, M.; Obara, H.; Suzuki, M.; Tanaka, M.; Fujioka, I.; et al. The potential failure risk of the cone-beam computed tomography-based planning target volume margin definition for prostate image-guided radiotherapy based on a prospective single-institutional hybrid analysis. *Radiat. Oncol.* **2018**, *13*, 106. [CrossRef]
50. Drozdz, S.; Schwedas, M.; Salz, H.; Foller, S.; Wendt, T.G. Prostate cancer treated with image-guided helical TomoTherapy and image-guided LINAC-IMRT. *Strahlenther. Onkol.* **2016**, *192*, 223–231. [CrossRef]
51. Rudat, V.; Nour, A.; Hammoud, M.; Alaradi, A.; Mohammed, A. Image-guided intensity modulated radiotherapy of prostate cancer. *Strahlenther. Onkol.* **2016**, *19*, 109–117. [CrossRef]
52. Chiesa, S.; Placidi, L.; Azario, L.; Mattiucci, G.C.; Greco, F.; Damiani, A.; Mantini, G.; Frascino, V.; Piermattei, A.; Valentini, V.; et al. Adaptive optimization by 6 DOF robotic couch in prostate volumetric IMRT treatment: Rototranslational shift and dosimetric consequences. *J. Appl. Clin. Med. Phys.* **2015**, *16*, 35–45. [CrossRef] [PubMed]
53. Li, M.; Li, G.F.; Hou, X.Y.; Gao, H.; Xu, Y.G.; Zhao, T.A. A dosimetric Comparison between Conventional Fractionated and Hypofractionated Image-guided Radiation Therapies for Localized Prostate Cancer. *Chin. Med. J.* **2016**, *129*, 1447–1454. [CrossRef] [PubMed]
54. Heng, S.P.; Low, S.H.; Sivamany, K. The influence of the bowel and bladder preparation protocol for radiotherapy of prostate cancer using kilo-voltage cone beam CT: Our experience. *Indian J. Cancer* **2015**, *52*, 639–644. [CrossRef] [PubMed]
55. Gozal, F.; Gondhowiardjo, S.A.; Kodrat, H.; Wibowo, W.E. Dosimetric analysis of three-dimensional conformal radiotherapy, intensity-modulated radiotherapy-step and shoot, helical tomotherapy, and volumetric modulated arc therapy in prostate cancer radiotherapy. *J. Cancer Res. Ther.* **2021**, *17*, 893–900. [CrossRef]
56. Pokhrel, D.; Tackett, T.; Stephen, J.; Visak, J.; Amin-Zimmerman, F.; McGregor, A.; Strup, S.E.; St Clair, W. Prostate SBRT using O-Ring Halcyon Linac. Plan quality, delivery efficiency, and accuracy. *J. Appl. Clin. Med. Phys.* **2020**, *22*, 68–75. [CrossRef]
57. Utsunomiya, S.; Yamamoto, J.; Tanabe, S.; Oishi, M.; Satsuma, A.; Kaidu, M.; Abe, E.; Ohta, A.; Kushima, N.; Aoyama, H. Complementary Relation Between the Improvement of Dose Delivery Technique and PTV Margin Reduction in Dose-Escalated Radiation Therapy for Prostate Cancer. *Pract. Radiat. Oncol.* **2019**, *9*, 172–178. [CrossRef]
58. Ma, T.M.; Ballas, L.K.; Wilhalme, H.; Sachdeva, A.; Chong, N.; Sharma, S.; Yang, T.; Basehart, V.; Reiter, R.E.; Saigal, C.; et al. Quality-of-Life Outcomes and Toxicity Profile Among Patients with Localized Prostate Cancer After Radical Prostatectomy Treated with Stereotactic Body Radiation: The SCIMITAR Multicenter Phase 2 Trial. *Int. J. Radiat. Oncol.* **2022**, *115*, 142–152. [CrossRef]
59. Walter, F.; Freislederer, P.; Belka, C.; Heinz, C.; Sohn, M.; Roeder, F. Evaluation of daily patient positioning for radiotherapy with a commercial 3D surface-imaging system (Catalyst). *Radiat. Oncol.* **2016**, *11*, 154. [CrossRef]
60. Batista, V.; Gober, M.; Moura, F.; Webster, A. Surface guided radiation therapy: An international survey on current clinical practice. *Tech. Innov. Patient Support. Radiat. Oncol.* **2022**, *22*, 1–8. [CrossRef]
61. Ariyaratne, H.; Chesham, H.; Pettingell, J.; Alonzi, R. Image-guided radiotherapy for prostate cancer with cone beam CT: Dosimetric effects of imaging frequency and PTV margin. *Radiother. Oncol.* **2016**, *121*, 103–108. [CrossRef]
62. Nichol, A.M.; Brock, K.K.; Lockwood, G.A. A magnetic resonance imaging study of prostate deformation relative to implanted gold fiducial markers. *Int. J. Radiat. Oncol. Biol. Phys.* **2017**, *67*, 48–56. [CrossRef]
63. Westley, L.R.; Alexander, S.E.; Goodwin, E. Magnetic resonance imageguided adaptive radiotherapy enables safe CTV-to-PTV margin reduction in prostate cancer: A cine MRI motion study. *Front. Oncol.* **2024**, *14*, 1379596. [CrossRef]
64. Onal, C.; Efe, E.; Bozca, R.; Yavas, C.; Yavas, G.; Arslan, G. The impact of margin reduction on radiation dose distribution of ultra-hypofractionated prostate radiotherapy utilizing a 1.5-T MR-Linac. *J. Appl. Clin. Med. Phys.* **2024**, *25*, e14179. [CrossRef] [PubMed]
65. *ICRU, Report 83*; Oxford University Press: Oxford, UK, 2010; Volume 10.
66. Moteabbed, M.; Trofimov, A.; Sharp, G.C.; Wang, Y.; Zietman, A.L.; Efstathiou, J.A.; Lu, H.M. A prospective comparison of the effects of interfractional variations on proton therapy and IMRT for prostate cancer. *Int. J. Rad. Oncol. Biol. Phys.* **2016**, *95*, 444–453. [CrossRef] [PubMed]
67. Maund, I.F.; Benson, J.; Fairfoul, J.; Cook, J.; Huddart, R.; Poynter, A. Image-guided radiotherapy of the prostate using daily CBCT: The feasibility and likely benefit of implementing a margin reduction. *Br. J. Radiol.* **2014**, *87*, 20140459. [CrossRef] [PubMed]
68. Dassen, M.G.; Janssen, T.; Kusters, M. Comparing adaptation strategies in MRI-guided online adaptive radiotherapy for prostate cancer: Implications for treatment margins. *Radiother. Oncol.* **2023**, *186*, 109761. [CrossRef]
69. Thome, W.D.; Paulsen, A. First experience and prospective evaluation on feasibility and acute toxicity of online adaptive radiotherapy of the prostate bed as salvage treatment in patients with biochemically recurrent prostate cancer on a 1.5T MR-linac. *J. Clin. Med.* **2022**, *11*, 4651.

70. Liu, L.; Wu, N.; Ouyang, H.; Dai, J.R.; Wang, W.H. Diffusion-weighted MRI in early assessment of tumour response to radiotherapy in high-risk prostate cancer. *Br. J. Radiol.* **2014**, *87*, 20140359. [CrossRef]
71. Künzel, L.A.; Leibfarth, S.; Dohm, O.S. Automatic VMAT planning for post-operative prostate cancer cases using particle swarm optimization: A proof of concept study. *Phys. Med.* **2020**, *69*, 101–109. [CrossRef]
72. Jeong, S.; Lee, J.H.; Chung, M.J.; Lee, S.W.; Lee, J.W.; Kang, D.G.; Kim, S.H. Analysis of Geometric Shifts and Proper Setup-Margin in Prostate Cancer Patients Treated With Pelvic Intensity-Modulated Radiotherapy Using Endorectal Ballooning and Daily Enema for Prostate Immobilization. *Medicine* **2016**, *95*, e2387. [CrossRef]
73. Knybel, L.; Cvek, J.; Blazek, T.; Binarova, A.; Parackova, T.; Resova, T. Prostate deformation during hypofractionated radiotherapy: An analysis of implanted fiducial marker displacement. *Radiat. Oncol.* **2021**, *16*, 235. [CrossRef] [PubMed]
74. Eminowicz, G.; Dean, C.; Shoffren, O.; Macdougall, N.; Wells, P.; Muirhead, R. Intensity modulated radiotherapy (IMRT) to prostate and pelvic nodes—Is pelvic lymph node coverage adequate with fiducial-based image-guided radiotherapy? *Br. J. Radiol.* **2014**, *87*, 20130696. [CrossRef] [PubMed]
75. Mahdavi, S.R.; Gharehbagh, E.J.; Mofid, B.; Jafari, A.H.; Nikoofar, A.R. Accuracy of the dose delivery in prostate cancer patients-using an electronic portal imaging device (EPID). *Int. J. Radiat. Res.* **2017**, *15*, 39–47.
76. Nourzadeh, H.; Watkins, W.T.; Ahmed, M.; Hui, C.; Schlesinger, D.; Siebersa, J.V. Clinical adequacy assessment of autocontours for prostate IMRT with meaningful endpoints. *Med. Phys.* **2017**, *44*, 1525–1537. [CrossRef]
77. Faccenda, V.; Panizza, D.; Daniotti, M.C.; Pellegrini, R.; Trivellato, S.; Caricato, P.; Lucchini, R.; De Ponti, E.; Arcangeli, S. Dosimetric Impact of Intrafraction Prostate Motion and Interfraction Anatomical Changes in Dose-Escalated Linac-Based SBRT. *Cancers* **2023**, *15*, 1153. [CrossRef]
78. Groher, M.; Kopp, P.; Drerup, M.; Deutschmann, H.; Sedlmayer, F.; Wolf, F. An IGRT margin concept for pelvic lymph nodes in high-risk prostate cancer. *Strahlenther. Onkol.* **2017**, *193*, 750–755. [CrossRef]
79. Willigenburg, T.; Zachiu, C.; Bol, G.H. Clinical application of a sub-fractionation workflow for intrafraction re-planning during prostate radiotherapy treatment on a 1.5 Tesla MR-Linac: A practical method to mitigate intrafraction motion. *Radiother. Oncol.* **2022**, *176*, 25–30. [CrossRef]
80. Van Nunen, A.; Van der Toorn, P.P.G.; Budiharto, T.C.G.; Schuring, D. Optimal image guided radiation therapy strategy for organs at risk sparing in radiotherapy of the prostate including pelvic lymph nodes. *Radiother. Oncol.* **2018**, *127*, 68–73. [CrossRef]
81. Arnaud, A.; Maingon, P.; Gauthier, M.; Naudy, S.; Dumas, J.; Martin, E.; Peignaux-Casasnovas, K.; Truc, G.; Bonnetain, F.; Crehange, G. Image guided IMRT for localized prostate cancer with daily repositioning: Inferring the difference between planned dose and delivered dose distribution. *Phys. Medica* **2014**, *30*, 669–675. [CrossRef]
82. Kasaova, L.; Sirak, M.; Jansa, J.; Paluska, P.; Petera, J. Quantitative Evaluation of the Benefit of Fiducial Image-Guidance for Prostate Cancer Intensity Modulated Radiation Therapy using Daily Dose Volume Histogram Analysis. *Technol. Cancer Res. Treat.* **2014**, *13*, 47–55. [CrossRef]
83. Onal, C.; Arslan, G.; Parlak, C.; Sonmez, S. Comparison of IMRT and VMAT plans with different energy levels using Monte-Carlo algorithm for prostate cancer. *Jpn. Radiol. Soc.* **2014**, *32*, 224–232. [CrossRef] [PubMed]
84. Park, J.M.; Park, S.Y.; Choi, C.H.; Chun, M.; Kim, J.H.; Kim, J.I. Treatment plan comparison between Tri-Co-60 magnetic resonance image-guided radiation therapy and volumetric modulated arc therapy for prostate cancer. *Oncotarget* **2017**, *8*, 91174–91184. [CrossRef]
85. Tøndel, H.; Lund, J.; Lydersen, S.; Wanderås, A.D.; Aksnessæther, B.; Jensen, C.A.; Kaasa, S.; Solberg, A. Radiotherapy for prostate cancer—Does daily image guidance with tighter margins improve patient reported outcomes compared to weekly orthogonal verified irradiation? Results from a randomized controlled trial. *Radiother. Oncol.* **2018**, *126*, 229–235. [CrossRef]
86. Scobioala, S.; Kittel, C.; Wissmann, N.; Haverkamp, U.; Channaoui, M.; Habibeh, O.; Elsayad, K.; Eich, H.T. A treatment planning study comparing tomotherapy, volumetric modulated arc therapy, Sliding Window and proton therapy for low-risk prostate carcinoma. *Radiat. Oncol.* **2016**, *11*, 128. [CrossRef]
87. Rossi, L.; Sharfo, A.W.; Aluwini, S.; Dirkx, M.; Breedveld, S.; Heijmen, B. First fully automated planning solution for robotic radiosurgery—Comparison with automatically planned volumetric arc therapy for prostate cancer. *Acta Oncol.* **2018**, *57*, 1490–1498. [CrossRef] [PubMed]
88. Wang, G.Y.; Zhu, Q.Z.; Zhu, H.L.; Jiang, L.J.; Zhao, N.; Liu, Z.K. Clinical performance evaluation of O-Ring Halcyon Linac: A realworld study. *World J. Clin. Cases* **2022**, *10*, 7728–7737. [CrossRef]
89. Bartlett, G.K.; Njeh, C.F.; Huang, K.C.; DesRosiers, C.; Guo, G. VMAT partial arc technique decreases dose to organs at risk in whole pelvic radiotherapy for prostate cancer when compared to full arc VMAT and IMRT. *Med. Dosim.* **2023**, *48*, 8–15. [CrossRef] [PubMed]
90. Fathy, M.M.; Hassan, B.Z.; El-Gebaly, H.R.; Mokhtar, M.H. Dosimetric evaluation study of IMRT and VMAT techniques for prostate cancer based on different multileaf collimator designs. *Radiat. Environ. Biophys.* **2023**, *62*, 97–106. [CrossRef]
91. Gao, L.R.; Tian, Y.; Wang, M.S. Assessment of delivered dose in prostate cancer patients treated with ultra-hypofractionated radiotherapy on 1.5-Tesla MR-Linac. *Front. Oncol.* **2023**, *13*, 1039901. [CrossRef]

92. Byrne, M.; Meei, A.Y.; Archibald-Heeren, B.; Hu, Y.; Rijken, J.; Luo, S.; Aland, T.; Greer, P. Intrafraction Motion and Margin Assessment for Ethos Online Adaptive Radiotherapy Treatments of the Prostate and Seminal Vesicles. *Adv. Radiat. Oncol.* **2024**, *9*, 101–405. [CrossRef]
93. Elith, C.A.; Dempsey, S.E.; Warren, H.M. Comparing four volumetric modulated arc therapy beam arrangements for the treatment of early-stage prostate cancer. *J. Med. Radiat. Sci.* **2014**, *61*, 91–101. [CrossRef] [PubMed]
94. Cakir, A.; Akgun, Z.; Fayda, M.; Agaoglu, M. Comparison of Three Dimensional Conformal Radiation Therapy, Intensity Modulated Radiation Therapy and Volumetric Modulated Arc Therapy for Low Radiation. *Asian Pac. J. Cancer Prev.* **2015**, *16*, 3365–3370. [CrossRef] [PubMed]
95. Oates, R.; Gill, S.; Foroudi, F.; Joon, M.L.; Schneider, M.; Bressel, M.; Kron, T. What benefit could be derived from on-line adaptive prostate radiotherapy using rectal diameter as a predictor of motion? *J. Med. Phys.* **2015**, *40*, 18–23. [CrossRef] [PubMed]
96. Yagihashi, T.; Inoue, K.; Nagata, H.; Yamanaka, M.; Yamano, A.; Suzuki, S.; Yamakabe, W.; Sato, N.; Omura, M.; Inoue, T. Effectiveness of robust optimization against geometric uncertainties in TomoHelical planning for prostate cancer. *J. Appl. Clin. Med. Phys.* **2023**, *24*, e13881. [CrossRef]
97. Polizzi, M.; Weiss, E.; Jan, N.; Ricco, A.; Kim, S.; Urdaneta, A.; Rosu-Bubulac, M. Rectal deformation management with IGRT in prostate radiotherapy: Can it be managed with rigid alignment alone. *J. Appl. Clin. Med. Phys.* **2024**, *25*, 14241. [CrossRef]

Current Oncology

MDPI

Systematic Review

A Meta-Analysis of Randomized Clinical Trials Assessing the Efficacy of PARP Inhibitors in Metastatic Castration-Resistant Prostate Cancer

Zakaria Alameddine [1,†], Muhammad Rafay Khan Niazi [1,†], Anisha Rajavel [1], Jai Behgal [1], Praneeth Reddy Keesari [1], Ghada Araji [1], Ahmad Mustafa [1], Chapman Wei [1], Abdullah Jahangir [2] and Terenig O Terjanian [1,*]

1 Staten Island University Hospital, Staten Island, NY 10305, USA; zalameddine@northwell.edu (Z.A.); mniazi@northwell.edu (M.R.K.N.); arajavel@northwell.edu (A.R.); jbehgal@northwell.edu (J.B.); pkeesari@northwell.edu (P.R.K.); garaji@northwell.edu (G.A.); amustafa3@northwell.edu (A.M.); cwei4@northwell.edu (C.W.)

2 University of Oklahoma Health Sciences Center, Oklahoma, OK 73104, USA; abdullah-jahangir@ouhsc.edu

* Correspondence: tterjanian@northwell.edu

† These authors contributed equally to this work.

Abstract: Prostate cancer ranks as the second most common malignancy in males. Prostate cancer progressing on androgen deprivation therapy (ADT) is castration-resistant prostate cancer (CRPC). Poly-ADP ribose polymerase (PARP) inhibitors (PARPis) have been at the forefront of the treatment of CRPC. We aim to better characterize the progression-free survival (PFS) and overall survival (OS) in metastatic CRPC patients treated with PARPis. A systemic review search was conducted using National Clinical Trial (NCT), PubMed, Embase, Scopus, and Central Cochrane Registry. The improvement in overall survival was statistically significant, favoring PARPis (hazard ratio (HR) 0.855; 95% confidence interval (CI) 0.752–0.974; $p = 0.018$). The improvement in progression-free survival was also statistically significant, with results favoring PARPis (HR 0.626; 95%CI 0.566–0.692; $p = 0.000$). In a subgroup analysis, similar results were observed where the efficacy of PARPis was evaluated in a subgroup of patients without homologous recombination repair (HRR) gene mutation, which showed improvement in PFS favoring PARPis (HR 0.747; 95%CI 0.0.637–0.877; $p = 0.000$). Our meta-analysis of seven RCTs showed that PARPis significantly increased PFS and OS when used with or without antihormonal agents like abiraterone or enzalutamide.

Keywords: castrate-resistant prostate cancer; PARP inhibitors; progression-free survival; overall survival; homologous recombination repair genes

1. Introduction

Prostate cancer ranks as the second most common malignancy in males and is estimated to be responsible for almost 5.5% of all cancer-related deaths in the United States [1,2]. Nevertheless, prognosis and treatment options for advanced disease remain complex [2,3].

Prostate cancer is classically driven by the accumulation of somatic and genetic mutations [1]. This is demonstrated by the higher risk of prostate cancer among the Ashkenazi Jewish population [1,2]. Mutations in genes involved with homologous recombination repair (HRR) are common in advanced prostate cancer, including *BRCA1* and *2* [1,2,4]. Targeting these mutations remains key to effectively treating advanced disease.

The Gleason Score, PSA level, PSA density, percentage of free PSA (free/total PSA ratio (f/t PSA)), and percentage of positive biopsy in core specimens determine the initial staging and prognosis of prostate cancer [2,3,5]. Depending on the life expectancy and symptoms of the patient, initial management for low-risk disease begins with active surveillance for progression [6,7]. The standard of care (SOC) for definitive treatment includes prostatectomy followed by radiation treatment [2,4,8]. Radiation options include external beam radiotherapy (EBRT) or brachytherapy [2]. In higher-risk diseases, radiation is followed by maintenance androgen-deprivation treatment (ADT) using gonadotropin-releasing hormone (GnRH) agonists and antagonists, with agents including leuprolide and goserelin [2,4].

Prostate cancer that progresses on ADT (for example, in the form of increased serum PSA, new metastasis, or progression of pre-existing metastasis) at castrate level testosterone level (<50 ng/dL) is termed castration-resistant prostate cancer (CRPC), and is characterized by changes in androgen receptor (AR) signaling [1,2,4]. CRPC requires additional hormone therapies such as apalutamide and enzalutamide [2,4]. Traditional chemotherapeutic agents, including docetaxel, etoposide, and platinum-based agents, are also used in the setting of metastatic CRPC [2,4,9]. PDL-1 inhibitors and cell therapies such as sipuleucel-T are also available [2,10,11]. In recent years, PARPis have been at the forefront of the treatment of CRPC. PARPis capitalize on mutations in homologous recombination repair (HRR) genes (such as *BRCA1* and 2, *ATM*), which are frequently found in CRPC [4,12].

PARPis have long been used in patients exhibiting *BRCA1* or 2 mutations in breast and ovarian cancers [13–16]. PARP1 is a protein that identifies and repairs single-strand breaks (SSBs) in DNA that have been subjected to oxidative stress [15,17,18]. Additionally, PARP1 functions alongside other proteins and via homologous recombination (HR) to repair damaged replication forks and restore DNA replication [17]. Doing so allows cancer cells to continue DNA synthesis and replication. The first PARPi for use in metastatic CRPC was approved by the FDA in 2020 [4].

Several trials have assessed the utility of PARPis in mCRPC [19–25]. Very recently, a meta-analysis that included Phase II/III studies comprising seventeen trials concluded that the benefit of PARPis was not uniform among the mCRPC patients and showed that the benefit was not uniformly spread between all the patients with alterations in DNA damage repair genes [26]. However, our study included only Phase III trials and showed the benefit of PARPis in improving radiologic PFS in patients with HRR gene alterations and patients lacking it. Previously, a meta-analysis by Niazi et al. that comprised three RCTs revealed significant survival benefits in patients with mCRPC who were treated with PARPis when compared to a placebo or traditional chemotherapies [4]. We performed this meta-analysis to improve the power of the study by Niazi et al., including additional clinical trials that have been performed to date. A subgroup analysis was performed to evaluate the results for patients without HRR gene mutation. The authors hypothesize that PARPis can be extended to a broader cancer population if supported by rigorous prospective trials. We aim to better characterize the progression-free survival (PFS) and overall survival (OS) in mCRPC patients treated with PARPis and determine the subgroup of patients with this disease who can benefit from these medications at maximum.

2. Methodology

The authors of this systematic review followed PRISMA guidelines and adhered to guidelines by the Cochrane Handbook for Systematic Reviews of Interventions in performing this analysis. The study protocol was not registered.

2.1. Search Strategy

The authors accessed Cochrane Central Registry of Clinical Trials, Embase, Scopus, NCT, and PubMed databases. MeSH (Medical Subject Heading) terms used were PARPi, Prostate cancer, Prostate neoplasm, Olaparib, rucaparib, veliparib, niraparib, talazoparib and docetaxel. The deadline for publication was set as 30 May 2023.

2.2. Inclusion and Exclusion Criteria

The papers included were as follows:

1. Randomized control trials comparing PARPis with or without androgen receptor pathway inhibitor (ARPI; abiraterone acetate or enzalutamide) against standard of care (ARPI or docetaxel) in prostate cancer patients;
2. Studies that reported progression-free survival and overall survival;
3. Patient age greater than 18 years;
4. Available in the English language without any restrictions on the date or status of the publication.

Papers that did not meet the above criteria were excluded.

2.3. Data Extraction

Information was extracted using a pre-specified extraction table. Information was filtered from trials through the reading of text and tables. Another author reviewed the information collected to ensure accuracy. The extracted data included Hazard ratios for progression-free survival and overall survival.

2.4. Trial Selection and Evaluation

Three authors independently reviewed all articles and abstracts and excluded the irrelevant trials. The risk of bias for selected papers was assessed using the Cochrane collaborative tool.

Based on this methodology, the risk of biases was classified into high, uncertain, and low (Figures 1 and 2).

2.5. Risk of Bias

Figures 1 and 2 exhibit the risk of bias.

2.6. Study Objectives

The objective of this analysis was to identify all the Phase III randomized controlled trials (RCTs) in which PARPis have been evaluated in the treatment of mCRPC and to compare the efficacy of PARPis among these patients with standard-of-care (SOC)/antihormonal therapies (abiraterone/enzalutamide) or chemotherapy in terms of progression-free survival (PFS) and overall survival (OS). We also aimed to perform an exploratory analysis on the subgroup of these patients who do not harbor HRR gene mutation to investigate the therapeutic efficacy of these agents in terms of PFS in this population.

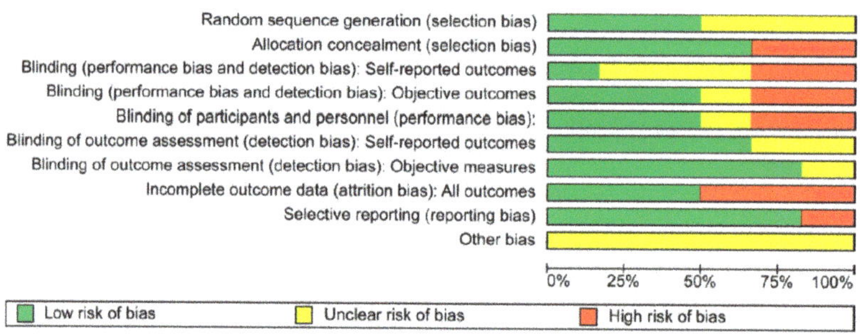

Figure 1. Risks of bias graph: review authors' judgment about each risk of bias item presented as percentages across all the included studies.

2.7. Statistical Analysis

Comprehensive Meta-Analysis software v. 3 was used to conduct this meta-analysis. Hazard ratios were calculated for PFS and overall survival. For effect sizes, 95%CI (confidence interval) was used, and for statistical significance, a p-value of less than 0.05 was used. Heterogeneity was evaluated using I^2 statistic, with heterogeneity less than 40 considered low, 40–60 considered moderate, and above 60 considered high. Where the median was used, it was assumed to be equivalent to the mean, and SD estimation was obtained by dividing the interquartile difference by 1.35. Fixed-effect analysis is usually adapted in cases where the I^2 value is ≤ 50; otherwise, a random-effect model is used.

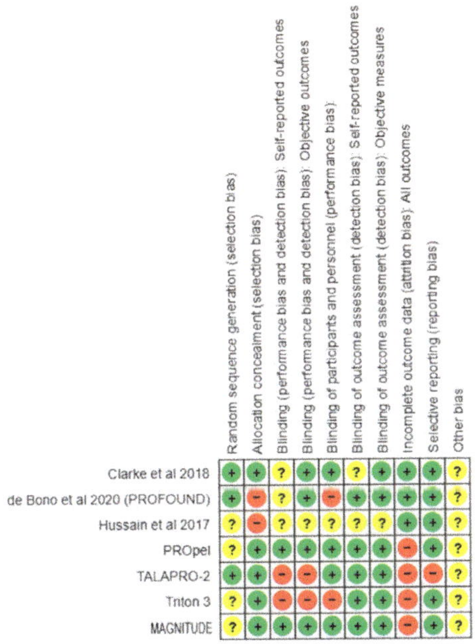

Figure 2. Risk of bias summary: review authors' judgment about each risk of bias item or each included study. Name of studies are mentioned along vertical axis. Whereas, characteristics are mentioned along horizontal axis. "+" denotes presence of each factor in the study; "−" denotes absence of that factor" and "?" means that it is uncertain [19–21].

3. Progression-Free Survival

3.1. Overview

The analysis was performed on all seven studies. The effect size index was the hazard ratio.

3.2. Statistical Model

Data were analyzed using a random-effect model since the studies were considered an arbitrary sample from a universe of all possible studies. This means that the results of this analysis can be generalized to the larger population of studies.

3.3. Mean Effect Size

The mean effect size was 0.630, with a 95% confidence interval of (0.547–0.726). This means we are 95% confident that the true mean effect size falls within this range in the universe of all comparable studies.

The Z-test was used to test the null hypothesis that the mean effect size is zero. The z-value was −6.415, with a p-value of <0.001. As a result, the null hypothesis can be rejected, and it can be concluded that the mean effect size in the universe of populations similar to those in the analysis is not zero.

3.4. Q-Test

The Q-statistic is a test of heterogeneity in meta-analysis. It tests the null hypothesis, which means all the studies included in the analysis have a common effect size. If this is true, then the expected value of the Q-statistic is equal to the degrees of freedom (df). In this analysis, the q-value was 10.971, with 6 df and $p = 0.089$. This means that the Q-statistic is significantly larger than the expected value, indicating heterogeneity among the studies. Using a criterion α of 0.100, the null hypothesis can be rejected. Hence, we can conclude that the studies do not share a common effect size.

3.5. The I^2 Statistic

The I^2 statistic of 45% indicates that 45% of the variation in the observed effects of the studies in the meta-analysis is due to variation in the true effects of the treatment in the different studies, rather than chance (sampling error).

4. Overall Survival

4.1. Overview

The analysis was performed on five out of the seven studies. The effect size index was the hazard ratio.

4.2. Statistical Model

This analysis was performed using the random-effect model. The studies included were considered an arbitrary sample from a universe of potential studies, and this analysis was utilized to make an inference to that universe.

4.3. Mean Effect Size

The mean effect size was 0.855, with a 95% confidence interval of (0.752–0.974). This means we are 95% confident that the true mean effect size falls within this range in the universe of all comparable studies. The Z-test was used to test the null hypothesis in which the mean effect size would be zero.

The z-value was -2.363, with a p-value of less than 0.018. As a result, the null hypothesis can be rejected, and it can be concluded that the mean effect size in the universe of populations similar to those in the analysis is not zero.

4.4. Q-Test

The Q-statistic is a test of heterogeneity in meta-analyses. It tests the null hypothesis which means all the studies included in the analysis have a common effect size. If this is true, then the expected value of the Q-statistic is equal to the degrees of freedom (df). The q-value was 2.888 with four degrees of freedom.

Since the q-value is less than the degrees of freedom, the amount of between-study variance in the observed effects is less than we expect based on sampling error alone. Therefore, true effect variance was estimated as zero, and all heterogeneity indices (I-squared, tau-squared, and tau) were set to zero.

4.5. The I^2 Statistic

The I^2 statistic of 0% indicates that 0% of the variation in the observed effects of the studies in the meta-analysis is due to variation in the true effects of the treatment in the different studies, rather than chance (sampling error).

5. Results

5.1. Study Selection and Characteristics

After the initial search, 494 articles were identified. Upon removing duplicates, 34 articles were shortlisted, and 406 were filtered out. The full text of 54 articles was analyzed. In total, 35 studies were identified as incomplete trials and hence precluded; 12 were review articles, 2 trials were terminated, 4 were single-arm studies, and 2 studies did not have a relevant intervention. Only seven randomized control trials were included, with 2688 patients. Figure 3 illustrates the PRISMA flow diagram.

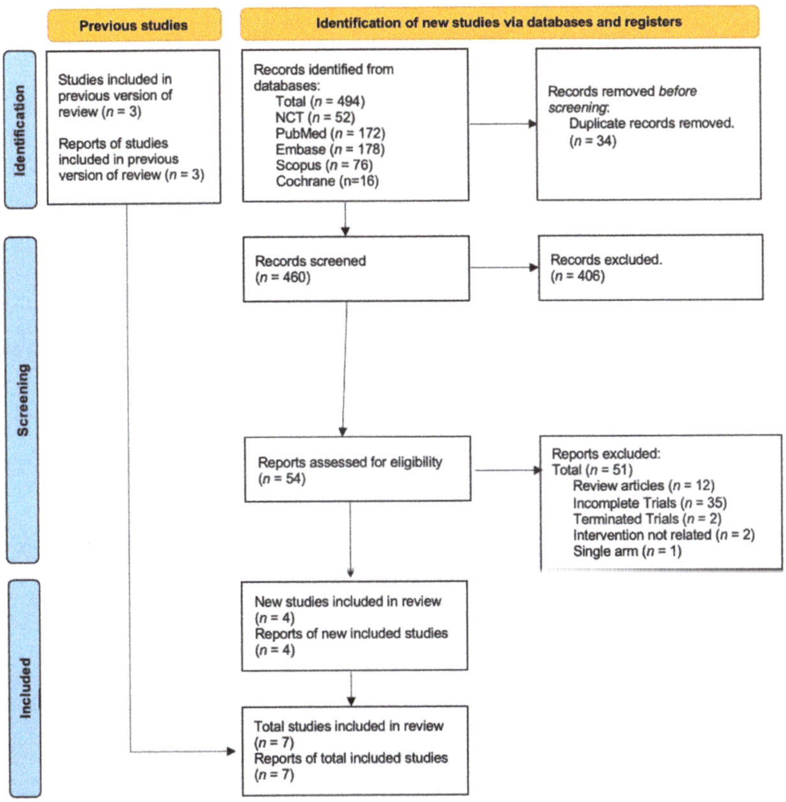

Figure 3. Prisma flow sheet diagram.

All seven studies used in this analysis were Phase III RCTs. Three of the trials used olaparib, whereas other studies used veliparib, rucaparib, niraparib, and talzoparib in the experimental arm against the standard-of-care treatment. Only four out of these seven studies reported the PFS outcomes for the subgroup of HRR wild-type patients, and that was used in the subgroup analysis. The main features of the included RCTs are listed in Table 1.

Table 1. Characteristics of randomized control trials (RCTs).

Study Name	Treatment Drugs	Study Characteristic	Inclusion	Exclusion	Primary Outcome
Clarke et al. (NCT01972217) [19]	olaparib (300 mg bid) + abiraterone (1000 mg/od) (*n* = 71) vs. abiraterone (1000 mg/od) alone (*n* = 71)	mCRPC patients previously treated with docetaxel and candidates for abiraterone treatment	Age >18 with mCRPC. ≤2 prior lines of chemotherapy, testosterone <50 ng/dL, no previous exposure to second-generation ARPI, candidates for abiraterone treatment, life expectancy ≥12 weeks, ECOG performance status of 0–2.	Previous treatment with PARPis, or cytotoxic chemotherapy. Other malignancies (including MGUS and MDS) within the last 5 years	Percentage of patients experiencing adverse events Number of patients with dose-limiting toxicities Median (rPFS) time percentage of patients with progression events or death

Table 1. *Cont.*

Study Name	Treatment Drugs	Study Characteristic	Inclusion	Exclusion	Primary Outcome
De Bono et al. PROfound study (NCT029 87543) [20]	olaparib (300 mg bid) vs. enzalutamide (160 mg/od) OR aberaterone (1000 mg/od) + Prednisone (5 mg/bid)	mCRPC patients with disease progression on treatment with enzalutamide or abiraterone Cohort A = Pts with at least one alteration in *BRCA1*, *BRCA2*, or *ATM* Cohort B = Pts with alteration in any of the other 12 genes	men (≥18 years of age) with mCRPC. ≤2 prior lines of chemotherapy, no previous exposure to second-generation antihormonal agents, candidates for abiraterone treatment, life expectancy ≥12 weeks, ECOG performance status of 0–2.	Previous treatment with PARPis, or cytotoxic chemotherapy. Other malignancies (including MGUS and MDS) within the last 5 years	PFS via RECIST (v1.1) for soft tissue, as a 20% increase in the sum of diameters of target lesions
Hussain et al. NCT01576172 [21].	Arm A = abiraterone (1000 mg) + prednisone (5 mg/bid) Arm B = veliparib (300 mg/bid)+ abiraterone (1000 mg) + prednisone (5 mg/bid)	pts stratified by ETS fusion status (positive or negative), randomly assigned to Arm (A) and (B)	Men with mCRPC, testosterone <50 ng/dL, ECOG status of 0 to 2, no prior exposure to abiraterone, and up to two prior chemotherapy regimens.	Chemotherapy, radiotherapy, history of active seizures, pituitary or adrenal dysfunction, active or symptomatic viral hepatitis, chronic liver disease, brain metastases	Confirmed PSA response rate time frame: up to 3 years
TRITON-3, NCT02975934	Arm A = oral rucaparib (600 mg twice daily). Arm B = physician's choice control (docetaxel or a second-generation ARPI (abiraterone acetate or enzalutamide))	Men with mCRPC and a BRCA or ATM alteration + disease progression on previous second-generation ARPI. Previous taxane-based chemotherapy for castration-sensitive disease was permitted.	men (≥18 years of age), with mCRPC, molecular evidence of *BRCA1/2* or *ATM* gene mutation. ECOG 0–1. Disease progression on prior ARPI	Active second malignancy, prior treatment with any PARPi, prior chemotherapy for mCRPC, metastasis to CNS	Assess the efficacy of rucaparib on the basis of rPFS in MCRPC patients with HRD who progressed on prior AR-directed therapy
Propel study NCT03732820	Arm A = oral abiraterone (1000 mg once daily) + olaparib (300 mg twice daily) + prednisone or prednisolone. Arm B = abiraterone + prednisolone + placebo	double-blind, randomized Phase III trial of abiraterone and olaparib versus abiraterone and placebo in first-line treatment of patients with mCRPC regardless of HRR status.	men (≥18 years of age), who are treatment naïve at mCRPC stage, ECOG 0–1, previous treatment with ARPI was allowed if it was at least 4 weeks before randomization	Active second malignancy, MDS or AML, prior treatment with any PARPi.	To determine the efficacy of the combination of olaparib and abiraterone vs. placebo and abiraterone by assessment of rPFS in patients with mCRPC who have received no prior cytotoxic chemotherapy or ARPI at mCRPC stage
TALAPRO-2 (NCT03395197)	Arm A = talazoparib 0.5 mg + enzalutamide 160 mg/daily, Arm B = placebo + enzalutamide 160 mg	pts randomized according to prior abiraterone or docetaxel for CSPC and HRR gene alteration status	Mildly or asymptomatic mCRPC with disease progression at study entry, ECOG PS ≤1, ongoing androgen deprivation therapy, no prior life-prolonging therapy for CRPC	Patients who received treatment at the CRPC stage, prior treatment with PARPis, ARPI, cytotoxic chemotherapy, Brain metastasis	To assess radiologic progression-free survival (rPFS) by BICR per RECIST (v.1.1)

Table 1. *Cont.*

Study Name	Treatment Drugs	Study Characteristic	Inclusion	Exclusion	Primary Outcome
MAGNI-TUDE TRIAL	niraparib 200 mg + abiraterone acetate 1000 mg plus prednisone 10 mg or placebo + AAP	Phase III, randomized, double-blind, placebo-controlled, multicenter study. The efficacy of Niraparib was assessed in HRR+ and HRR-negative patients	Pt who had used ARPI for less than 4 months, prior systemic therapy (docetaxel, enzalutamide, apalutamide, darolutamide) for metastatic castration-sensitive prostate cancer or non-metastatic castration-resistant prostate cancer. No prior use of PARPis	Prior use of PARPis, Use of AAP more than 2–4 months prior to randomization, History of CAD, brain metastasis, or MDS/AML	To evaluate the effectiveness of niraparib and AAP compared to AAP and placebo, as determined by radiographic progression-free survival (rPFS)

ARPI—androgen receptor pathway inhibitor; AR—androgen receptor; HRR—homologous recombination repair; mCRPC—metastatic castration-resistant prostate cancer; ECOG—eastern cooperative oncology group; PARPis—poly(adenosine diphosphate ribose) polymerase inhibitors; MDS—myelodysplastic syndrome; MGUS—monoclonal gammopathy of undetermined significance; rPFS—radiologic progression-free survival; RECIST (v1.1)—response evaluation criteria in solid tumors; PSA—prostate-specific antigen.

5.2. Quality of Studies

Cochrane's risk of bias tools determined the risk of bias in each study. The "risk of bias graph" shows that the study had a low risk for selection bias secondary to random sequence generation and allocation concealment. Furthermore, studies were double-blinded, decreasing the risk of performance and detection bias. Overall, a low to moderate risk of bias in the studies suggests that the results of this meta-analysis may be subjected to bias. However, the results are still likely to be reliable, as they are based on many studies.

5.3. Result of Quantitative Analysis

5.3.1. Overall Survival (OS)

Five studies [19,20,22–24] reported overall survival when using PARPis compared with standard of care. The pooled results showed that PFS was significantly better with PARPis (hazard ratio (HR) = 0.855; 95%CI 0.752–0.974; $p = 0.018$) (Figure 4). The pooled analysis was homogeneous ($I^2 = 0\%$, q-value 2.888 with 4 df), and a fixed-effect model was used.

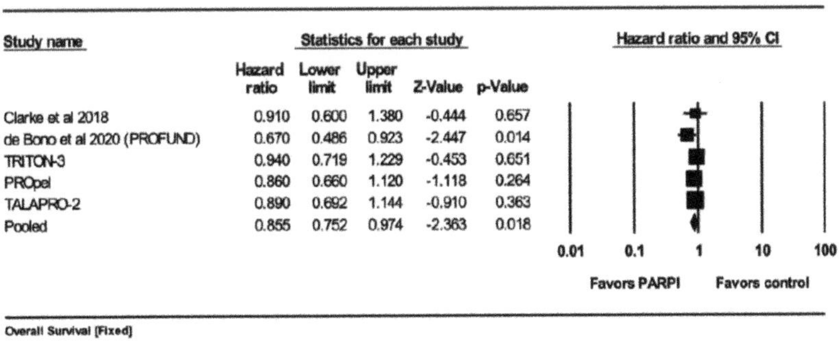

Figure 4. Forrest plot for comparing the overall survival using a fixed-effect model. The mean effect size was 0.855 with a 95% confidence interval of 0.752 to 0.974. The z-value was -2.363 with $p = 0.018$. The I-squared statistic was 0% [19,20].

5.3.2. Progression-Free Survival (PFS)

Seven studies [19–25] reported progression-free survival when using PARPis compared with standard of care. The improvement in progression-free survival was found to be statistically significant and favored PARPis (HR 0.626; 95%CI 0.566–0.692; p = 0.000). The pooled analysis was homogeneous (I^2 = 45% and q-test for heterogeneity; p-value = 0.089), and a fixed-effect model was used (Figure 5).

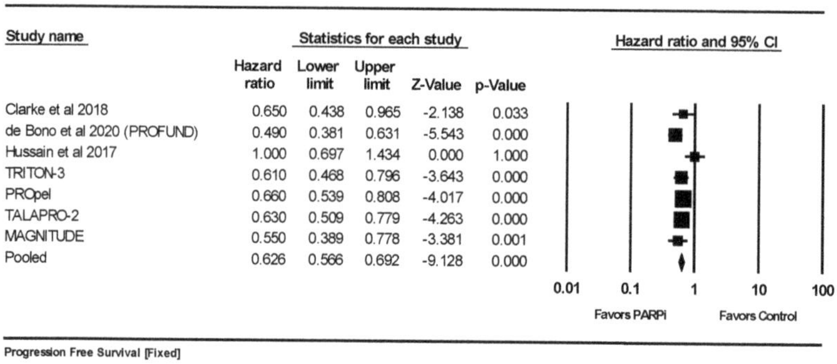

Figure 5. Forrest plot for comparing the progression-free survival using a fixed-effect model. The mean effect size was 0. 626 with a 95% confidence interval between 0.566 and 0.692 with a z-value of −9.128 and a p-value = 0.000. The improvement in progression-free survival was statistically significant [19–21].

5.3.3. Progression-Free Survival (PFS) in Patients without HRR Gene Mutation

Four studies reported progression-free survival when using PARPis compared with standard of care in a subgroup of patients without HRR gene mutation. The results favored PARPis (HR 0.747; 95%CI 0.0.637–0.877; p = 0.000), and I^2 = 0 (Figure 6).

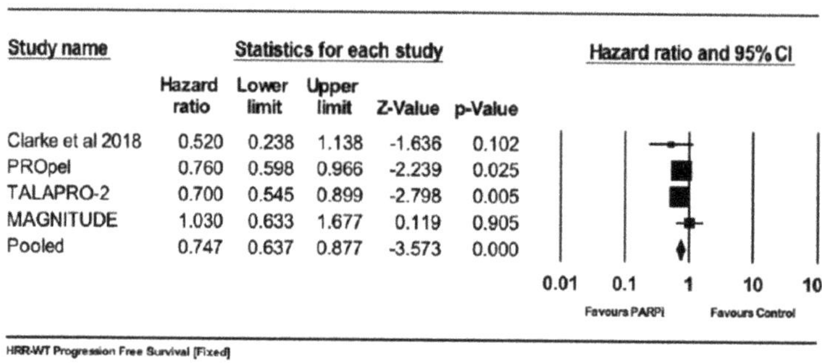

Figure 6. Forrest plot for comparing the progression-free survival in the subgroup of patients without HRR gene mutation. The effect size was 0.747 with a 95% confidence interval between 0.637 and 0.877, with a z-value of −3.573, a p-value = 0.000, and an I-squared statistics = 0. The results favored PARPis [19].

6. Discussion

Prostate cancer remains the second most common malignancy in males [2]. Current SOC treatment includes prostatectomy, radiation, and ADT [2]. Progression on ADT is termed castration resistance and treatment for metastatic castration-resistant prostate cancer (mCRPC) is less defined [2]. Recently, PARPis have been under investigation to treat mCRPC as monotherapy in second- or third-line treatment options.

Our meta-analysis of clinical trials revealed that PARPis may improve both PFS (HR 0.626, 95%CI 0.566–0.692, p = 0.000) and OS (HR 0.855, 95%CI 0.752–0.974, p = 0.018) in patients with mCRPC as compared to placebo or SOC chemotherapy or ADT. These results were computed using the fixed-effect model. The findings also held true using the random-effect model. Moreover, when a subgroup analysis was performed for the patient population who lacked HRR gene mutation, PFS was improved, favoring PARPis (HR 0.747 (0.0.637–0.877), $p = 0.000$) and $I^2 = 0$.

Two PARPis were initially FDA-approved for use in mCRPC in 2020: Rucaparib was approved for use in mCRPC with somatic and/or germline *BRCA1* or *BRCA2* mutations based on TRITON2 [27], and olaparib was approved for mCRPC with HRR gene mutations based on the PROfound trial [20]. So far, as per the NCCN guidelines and FDA approval of rucaparib and olaparib, they are not used as first-line treatment for mCRPC either alone or in combination with ADT. Overall, three trials (BRCAAWAY, MAGNITUDE, and PROPEL) showed improvement in the PFS with PARPis (olaparib, niraparib, and olaparib, respectively) when used in combination with ADT as the first-line treatment for mCRPC, but there was no survival benefit [24,25,28]. Similarly, the results for this combination for patients previously treated with ADT with or without chemotherapy are promising, but it is not recommended outside the clinical trial by NCCN. Numerous other RCTs are currently underway studying the efficacy of PARPis including olaparib, veliparib, rucaparib, niraparib (Zejula), and talazoparib (Talzenna) with and without ADT in mCRPC. Our search of www.clinicaltrials.gov (accessed on 30 May 2023) revealed approximately 39 RCTs studying PARPis in prostate cancer: 19 actively recruiting, 10 completed or nearly completed, and 7 trials with results.

Three trials investigated the efficacy of olaparib. The first two trials were carried out by Clarke et al. [19] and de Bono et al. [20]. PARPis are effective in mCRPC patients irrespective of the genetic mutation status. However, the analysis performed later by reconstructing the data from the original study revealed that patients in Cohort B (those without HRR genetic alteration) failed to derive any PFS benefit [29]. The study by Clarke et al. aimed to show the benefit of PARPis and novel hormonal agent synergy across all the mCRPC patients regardless of HRR mutation status. Authors hypothesized that the combination of PARPis and novel hormonal agents could be effective in HRR wild-type patients because androgen receptors regulate DNA transcription, and PARP enzyme is used in this process that PARPis can target. Secondly, androgen depletion impairs HRR, producing a BRCA-like phenotype susceptible to PARP inhibition [19]. The third trial is the PROpel study (NCT03732820) [24]. Patients who failed primary androgen deprivation therapy were randomized into those receiving abiraterone and either olaparib or placebo irrespective of HRR mutation status. The study showed significant prolongation in PFS in the treatment group at 24.8 months vs. 16.6 months in the control group (HR 0.66, 95%CI, [0.54–0.81]; $p < 0.0001$). These results exhibit the prospects of PARPis in a broader population of patients with mCRPC, irrespective of HRR mutation status, who have failed earlier line treatment. The overall survival benefit was not significant in this study. Nevertheless, the study results have not matured yet (data maturity: 28.6%).

The fourth trial investigated the efficacy of veliparib (NCT01576172; Hussain et al.) [21] against the standard of care (abiraterone plus prednisone). The major goal of this trial was to investigate whether ETS fusion status (family of transcription factors) had any effect on tumor response to treatment. Patients were divided into case and control cohorts equally after being classified as having an ETS fusion or not (positive or negative). PFS was found to be similar in both treatment arms. PFS in the treatment group was 11 months (95%CI, 8.1–13.6) vs. 10.1 months (95%CI, 8.2–13.8) in the control group ($p = 0.99$).

The efficacy of rucaparib was originally demonstrated in the Triton-2 trial [27], the results of which were later verified in a Phase III trial (Triton-3) [23]. Patients enrolled in this trial had mCRPC with a *BRCA1*, *BRCA2*, or *ATM* mutation with disease progression after ADT treatment. They were randomly divided into two groups, one receiving rucaparib and the other docetaxel or ADT (abiraterone or enzalutamide). Compared with the previous studies, this was the first study where patients received chemotherapy in the SOC group. The population in the intention-to-treat group comprised patients who had undergone randomization, with a prespecified subgroup of BRCA-mutated patients. There was a significant improvement in the rucaparib group in comparison to the control group in the

BRCA analysis and the intention-to-treat (ITT) analysis in BRCA subgroup: 11.2 months (CI, 9.2 to 13.8) vs. 6.4 months (CI, 5.4 to 8.3) (HR, 0.50; 95%CI, 0.36 to 0.69; $p < 0.001$ by log-rank test); in ITT group, patients with the BRCA mutation had greater benefits than those with the ATM mutation. The overall survival benefit was not significant in this study. Nevertheless, the study results have not matured yet (data maturity: 54%).

Agarwal et al. studied the efficacy of talazoparib, a PARPi that was approved for the treatment of locally advanced or metastatic breast cancer harboring a BRCA mutation, in patients with mCRPC [22]. In TALAPRO-2 (NCT03395197) [22], patients were randomized to receive enzalutamide either with talazoparib or with a placebo. Patients enrolled in this study had disease progression while on androgen deprivation therapy. The results of this study showed a significant improvement in PFS in HRR-deficient (HR, 0.46; 95%CI, 0.30–0.70; $p < 0.001$), HRR-non-deficient or unknown (HR, 0.70; 95%CI, 0.54–0.89; $p = 0.004$), and HRR-non-deficient patients based on tumor tissue testing (HR, 0.66; 95%CI, 0.49–0.91; $p = 0.009$). Hence, this indicates that the addition of talazoparib on enzalutamide had significant improvement in PFS over enzalutamide alone (considered the standard of care) in patients with mCRPC regardless of HRR status.

The MAGNITUDE trial [25] was a placebo–control study where niraparib was combined with abiraterone and prednisone in the experimental arm and compared with abiraterone/prednisone plus placebo. Patients could have received systemic therapies before enrollment for non-metastatic prostate cancer or metastatic castration-resistant prostate cancer. This study also showed a 45% reduction in rPFS or death. The overall survival data were not immature at the time of publication. In this trial, rPFS was evaluated in the HRR+ cohort with subgroup analysis of *BRCA1*/2-positive patients. A futility analysis for HRR patients was also performed with PARPis, which confirmed no benefit from medication in this population.

Another interesting finding in this study was the subgroup analysis performed on the patients without HRR gene mutation. Out of the seven studies, only four reported the efficacy of the PARPis in terms of PFS in this patient population. The subgroup analysis showed statistically significant improvement in the PFS of this patient population (HR 0.719 (0.607–0.852), $p = 0.000$), an effect that was previously endorsed by the TALAPRO-2 and PROPEL study. These results favor the utility of PARPis in patients with mCRPC regardless of HRR gene mutation status and encourage trials to target a broader patient population who can benefit from the synergy of PARPis and novel antihormonal agents. Authors hypothesized that the combination of PARPis and novel hormonal agents could be effective in HRR wild-type patients because androgen receptors regulate DNA transcription, and PARP enzyme is used in this process that PARPis can target. Hence, the inhibition of the PARP pathway enhances the antiandrogenic effect by suppressing the androgen receptor's transcription. Secondly, androgen depletion impairs HRR, producing a BRCA-like phenotype susceptible to PARP inhibition [19,30,31].

In contrast to previous studies, the results we observed can translate to meaningful improvement in the overall and progression-free survival in patients with mCRPC. Although the effect was enhanced in the patients who harbored genetic mutations in HRR genes, it still shows a significant improvement in the PFS among patients without HRR gene mutations. In recent RCTs, PARPi was used as a second-line treatment even before chemotherapy and was shown to have promising results. The results of this metanalysis favor the use of PARPis in combination with novel hormonal agents like enzalutamide and abiraterone, regardless of their HRR alterations status, with an acceptable side-effect profile. Additionally, this analysis encourages the consideration of using this combination in upfront treatments for mCRPC rather than in second- or third-line treatment options in which this drug combo can be utilized in a broader population than the patient population currently seen in our clinics who have the potential to derive survival benefits from it.

Strengths and Limitations

We acknowledge several limitations to this study. These include limited availability of Phase II and III RCTs, as well as the lack of heterogeneity in patient population and narrow inclusionary criteria of patients. Data were derived from only seven studies at the study level, not the patient level. Since the total number of studies was less than 10, publication bias could not be reliably ruled out, which can lead to an overestimation of the results. This can be minimized by including more clinical trials when their results are published. This requires close circumspection while applying the results to the general population. The overall survival data from the newer studies have yet to mature and would require a follow-up of these studies to reanalyze the data. Therefore, the results of this analysis need to be interpreted with caution. Lastly, the study protocol was not registered. Future studies that assess the adverse effects of the medications used in the RCTs would be beneficial. The primary strength of this meta-analysis is that it encompasses all the completed Phase III RCTs.

7. Conclusions

Our meta-analysis of clinical trials found that PARPis in combination with novel hormonal agents may improve both progression-free survival (PFS) and overall survival (OS) in patients with metastatic castration-resistant prostate cancer (mCRPC), regardless of their HRR gene mutation status.

These findings suggest that PARPis in combination with novel hormonal agents may be a promising new treatment option for patients with mCRPC, even in patients who do not have HRR gene mutations. This is a significant finding, as it could expand the number of patients who are eligible for PARPi therapy.More research is needed to confirm these findings and to determine the optimal use of PARPis in combination with novel hormonal agents for the treatment of mCRPC.

Author Contributions: Z.A., M.R.K.N., A.R., J.B., G.A. and P.R.K. were behind the conceptualization of the main idea. Z.A., M.R.K.N., A.R. and G.A. were involved in writing original draft. A.M., A.J. and C.W. with formal analaysis and using the software. J.B and P.R.K. helped with data curation. T.O.T. and M.R.K.N. were involved in Supervision, visualization and writing (review and editing). All authors have read and agreed to the published version of the manuscript.

Funding: This research received no external funding.

Acknowledgments: We would like to thank the editors of "Current Oncology" for their time and consideration in reviewing this manuscript. We are grateful for their helpful feedback and suggestions, which have helped us to improve the quality of our work.

Conflicts of Interest: The authors declare no conflict of interest.

References

1. Rebello, R.J.; Oing, C.; Knudsen, K.E. Prostate cancer. *Nat. Rev. Dis. Primers* **2021**, *7*, 8.
2. Barsouk, A.; Padala, S.A.; Vakiti, A.; Mohammed, A.; Saginala, K.; Thandra, K.C.; Barsouk, A. Epidemiology, Staging and Management of Prostate Cancer. *Med. Sci.* **2020**, *8*, 28.
3. Welch, H.G.; Albertsen, P.C. Reconsidering Prostate Cancer Mortality—The Future of PSA Screening. *N. Engl. J. Med.* **2020**, *382*, 1557–1563. [PubMed]
4. Niazi, M.R.K.; Jahangir, A.; Sahra, S.; Sattar, S.B.A.; Asti, D.; Bershadskiy, A. Efficacy of PARP Inhibitors as Maintenance Therapy for Metastatic Castration-Resistant Prostate Cancer: A Meta-Analysis of Randomized Controlled Trials. *Oncology* **2021**, *35*, 708–715. [PubMed]
5. Ferraro, S.; Biganzoli, G.; Bussetti, M.; Castaldi, S.; Biganzoli, E.M.; Plebani, M. Managing the impact of inter-method bias of prostate specific antigen assays on biopsy referral: The key to move towards precision health in prostate cancer management. *Clin. Chem. Lab. Med.* **2023**, *61*, 142–153. [PubMed]
6. Ng, S.P.; Duchesne, G.; Tai, K.-H.; Foroudi, F.; Kothari, G.; Williams, S. Support for the use of objective comorbidity indices in the assessment of noncancer death risk in prostate cancer patients. *Prostate Int.* **2017**, *5*, 8–12. [PubMed]
7. Cooperberg, M.R.; Carroll, P.R.; Klotz, L. Active Surveillance for Prostate Cancer: Progress and Promise. *J. Clin. Oncol.* **2011**, *29*, 3669–3676. [PubMed]

8. Wolff, R.F.; Ryder, S.; Bossi, A.; Briganti, A.; Crook, J.; Henry, A.; Karnes, J.; Potters, L.; de Reijke, T.; Stone, N.; et al. A systematic review of randomised controlled trials of radiotherapy for localised prostate cancer. *Eur. J. Cancer* **2015**, *51*, 2345–2367.
9. Corn, P.G.; I Heath, E.; Zurita, A.; Ramesh, N.; Xiao, L.; Sei, E.; Li-Ning-Tapia, E.; Tu, S.-M.; Subudhi, S.K.; Wang, J.; et al. Cabazitaxel plus carboplatin for the treatment of men with metastatic castration-resistant prostate cancers: A randomised, open-label, phase 1–2 trial. *Lancet Oncol.* **2019**, *20*, 1432–1443.
10. Rathi, N.; McFarland, T.R.; Nussenzveig, R.; Agarwal, N.; Swami, U. Evolving Role of Immunotherapy in Metastatic Castration Refractory Prostate Cancer. *Drugs* **2021**, *81*, 191–206.
11. Garcia, J.A. Sipuleucel-T in patients with metastatic castration-resistant prostate cancer: An insight for oncologists. *Ther. Adv. Med. Oncol.* **2011**, *3*, 101–108. [CrossRef]
12. Wu, K.; Liang, J.; Shao, Y.; Xiong, S.; Feng, S.; Li, X. Evaluation of the Efficacy of PARP Inhibitors in Metastatic Castration-Resistant Prostate Cancer: A Systematic Review and Meta-Analysis. *Front. Pharmacol.* **2021**, *12*, 777663. [CrossRef]
13. Wang, S.S.Y.; Jie, Y.E.; Cheng, S.W.; Ling, G.L.; Ming, H.V.Y. PARP Inhibitors in Breast and Ovarian Cancer. *Cancers* **2023**, *15*, 2357. [CrossRef] [PubMed]
14. Shao, F.; Duan, Y.; Zhao, Y.; Li, Y.; Liu, J.; Zhang, C.; He, S. PARP inhibitors in breast and ovarian cancer with BRCA mutations: A meta-analysis of survival. *Aging* **2021**, *13*, 8975–8988. [CrossRef] [PubMed]
15. Sugimura, K.; Takebayashi, S.-I.; Taguchi, H.; Takeda, S.; Okumura, K. PARP-1 ensures regulation of replication fork progression by homologous recombination on damaged DNA. *J. Cell Biol.* **2008**, *183*, 1203–1212. [CrossRef] [PubMed]
16. Konecny, G.E.; Kristeleit, R.S. PARP inhibitors for BRCA1/2-mutated and sporadic ovarian cancer: Current practice and future directions. *Br. J. Cancer* **2016**, *115*, 1157–1173. [CrossRef]
17. Slade, D. PARP and PARG inhibitors in cancer treatment. *Genes. Dev.* **2020**, *34*, 360–394. [CrossRef]
18. Pham, M.M.; Ngoi, N.Y.; Peng, G.; Tan, D.S.; Yap, T.A. Development of poly(ADP-ribose) polymerase inhibitor and immunotherapy combinations: Progress, pitfalls, and promises. *Trends Cancer* **2021**, *7*, 958–970. [CrossRef]
19. Clarke, N.; Wiechno, P.; Alekseev, B.; Sala, N.; Jones, R.; Kocak, I.; Chiuri, V.E.; Jassem, J.; Fléchon, A.; Redfern, C. {Rebello, 2021 #22}{Rebello, 2021 #22} Olaparib combined with abiraterone in patients with metastatic castration-resistant prostate cancer: A randomised, double-blind, placebo-controlled, phase 2 trial. *Lancet Oncol.* **2018**, *19*, 975–986.
20. de Bono, J.; Mateo, J.; Fizazi, K.; Saad, F.; Shore, N.; Sandhu, S.; Hussain, M. Olaparib for Metastatic Castration-Resistant Prostate Cancer. *N. Engl. J. Med.* **2020**, *382*, 2091–2102. [CrossRef]
21. Hussain, M.; Daignault-Newton, S.; Twardowski, P.W.; Albany, C.; Stein, M.N.; Kunju, L.P.; Chinnaiyan, A.M. Targeting Androgen Receptor and DNA Repair in Metastatic Castration-Resistant Prostate Cancer: Results From NCI 9012. *J. Clin. Oncol.* **2018**, *36*, 991–999. [CrossRef]
22. Agarwal, N.; Azad, A.; Carles, J.; Fay, A.P.; Matsubara, N.; Heinrich, D.; Szczylik, C.; De Giorgi, U.; Joung, J.Y.; Fong, P.C.; et al. TALAPRO-2: Phase 3 study of talazoparib (TALA) + enzalutamide (ENZA) versus placebo (PBO) + ENZA as first-line (1L) treatment in patients (pts) with metastatic castration-resistant prostate cancer (mCRPC). *J. Clin. Oncol.* **2023**, *41* (Suppl. S6), LBA17. [CrossRef]
23. Fizazi, K.; Piulats, J.M.; Reaume, M.N.; Ostler, P.; McDermott, R.; Gingerich, J.R.; Pintus, E.; Sridhar, S.S.; Bambury, R.M.; Emmenegger, U.; et al. Rucaparib or Physician's Choice in Metastatic Prostate Cancer. *N. Engl. J. Med.* **2023**, *388*, 719–732. [CrossRef]
24. Saad, F.; Armstrong, A.J.; Thiery-Vuillemin, A.; Oya, M.; Loredo, E.; Procopio, G.; de Menezes, J.J.; Girotto, G.C.; Arslan, C.; Mehra, N.; et al. PROpel: Phase III trial of olaparib (ola) and abiraterone (abi) versus placebo (pbo) and abi as first-line (1L) therapy for patients (pts) with metastatic castration-resistant prostate cancer (mCRPC). *J. Clin. Oncol.* **2022**, *40* (Suppl. S6), 11. [CrossRef]
25. Chi, K.; Sandhu, S.; Smith, M.; Attard, G.; Saad, M.; Olmos, D.; Castro, E.; Roubaud, G.; Gomes, A.P.d.S.; Small, E.; et al. Niraparib plus abiraterone acetate with prednisone in patients with metastatic castration-resistant prostate cancer and homologous recombination repair gene alterations: Second interim analysis of the randomized phase III MAGNITUDE trial. *Ann. Oncol.* **2023**, *34*, 772–782. [CrossRef]
26. Iannantuono, G.M.; Chandran, E.; Floudas, C.S.; Choo-Wosoba, H.; Butera, G.; Roselli, M.; Gulley, J.L.; Karzai, F. Efficacy and safety of PARP inhibitors in metastatic castration-resistant prostate cancer: A systematic review and meta-analysis of clinical trials. *Cancer Treat Rev.* **2023**, *120*, 102623. [CrossRef] [PubMed]
27. Abida, W.; Patnaik, A.; Campbell, D.; Shapiro, J.; Bryce, A.H.; McDermott, R.; Sautois, B.; Vogelzang, N.J.; Bambury, R.M.; Voog, E.; et al. Rucaparib in Men with Metastatic Castration-Resistant Prostate Cancer Harboring a BRCA1 or BRCA2 Gene Alteration. *J. Clin. Oncol.* **2020**, *38*, 3763–3772. [CrossRef]
28. Hussain, M.H.A.; Kocherginsky, M.; Agarwal, N.; Zhang, J.; Adra, N.; Paller, C.J.; Picus, J.; Reichert, Z.R.; Szmulewitz, R.Z.; Tagawa, S.T.; et al. BRCAAWAY: A randomized phase 2 trial of abiraterone, olaparib, or abiraterone + olaparib in patients with metastatic castration-resistant prostate cancer (mCRPC) with DNA repair defects. *J. Clin. Oncol.* **2022**, *40* (Suppl. S16), 5018. [CrossRef]
29. Stopsack, K.H. Efficacy of PARP Inhibition in Metastatic Castration-resistant Prostate Cancer is Very Different with Non-BRCA DNA Repair Alterations: Reconstructing Prespecified Endpoints for Cohort B from the Phase 3 PROfound Trial of Olaparib. *Eur. Urol.* **2021**, *79*, 442–445. [CrossRef] [PubMed]

30. Congregado, B.; Rivero, I.; Osmán, I.; Sáez, C.; López, R.M. PARP Inhibitors: A New Horizon for Patients with Prostate Cancer. *Biomedicines* **2022**, *10*, 1416. [CrossRef] [PubMed]
31. Asim, M.; Tarish, F.; Zecchini, H.I.; Sanjiv, K.; Gelali, E.; Massie, C.E.; Baridi, A.; Warren, A.Y.; Zhao, W.; Ogris, C.; et al. Synthetic lethality between androgen receptor signalling and the PARP pathway in prostate cancer. *Nat. Commun.* **2017**, *8*, 374. [CrossRef] [PubMed]

Current Oncology

MDPI

Communication

Review on the Role of BRCA Mutations in Genomic Screening and Risk Stratification of Prostate Cancer

Nikolaos Kalampokis [1], Christos Zabaftis [2], Theodoros Spinos [3], Markos Karavitakis [2], Ioannis Leotsakos [2], Ioannis Katafigiotis [2], Henk van der Poel [4], Nikolaos Grivas [2,4,*] and Dionysios Mitropoulos [5]

1 Department of Urology, G. Hatzikosta General Hospital, 45001 Ioannina, Greece; kalampokas88@gmail.com
2 Department of Laparoscopy and Endourology, Central Urology, Lefkos Stavros the Athens Clinic, PC 11528 Athens, Greece; zabaftisc@gmail.com (C.Z.); markoskaravitakis@yahoo.gr (M.K.); ioannisdleotsakos@gmail.com (I.L.); katafigiotis.giannis@gmail.com (I.K.)
3 Department of Urology, University of Patras Hospital, 26504 Patras, Greece; thspinos@otenet.gr
4 Department of Urology, The Netherlands Cancer Institute-Antoni van Leeuwenhoek Hospital, 1066 CX Amsterdam, The Netherlands; h.vd.poel@nki.nl
5 Department of Urology, Medical School, National & Kapodistrian University of Athens, 14122 Athens, Greece; dmitrop@med.uoa.gr
* Correspondence: nikolaosgrivas@hotmail.com; Tel.: +31-205121543; Fax: +31-205122459

Abstract: (1) Background: Somatic and germline alterations can be commonly found in prostate cancer (PCa) patients. The aim of our present study was to perform a comprehensive review of the current literature in order to examine the impact of BRCA mutations in the context of PCa as well as their significance as genetic biomarkers. (2) Methods: A narrative review of all the available literature was performed. Only "landmark" publications were included. (3) Results: Overall, the number of PCa patients who harbor a BRCA2 mutation range between 1.2% and 3.2%. However, BRCA2 and BRCA1 mutations are responsible for most cases of hereditary PCa, increasing the risk by 3–8.6 times and up to 4 times, respectively. These mutations are correlated with aggressive disease and poor prognosis. Gene testing should be offered to patients with metastatic PCa, those with 2–3 first-degree relatives with PCa, or those aged < 55 and with one close relative with breast (age $\leq$ 50 years) or invasive ovarian cancer. (4) Conclusions: The individualized assessment of BRCA mutations is an important tool for the risk stratification of PCa patients. It is also a population screening tool which can guide our risk assessment strategies and achieve better results for our patients and their families.

Keywords: prostate cancer; genomic screening; mutations

1. Introduction

Based on epidemiological data, prostate cancer (PCa) has been shown to be the most common of all urologic malignancies and second only to lung cancer as regards cancer-related mortality among male patients in developed countries [1]. The incidence of the disease has been steadily increasing over recent years [2], with the lifetime risk being equal to 12%, while the median age of diagnosis is 66 years according to the SEER database [3]. Although the widespread use of PSA as a screening tool has markedly increased the number of patients being diagnosed with occult disease [4], early detection has substantially decreased both cancer-specific mortality and advanced disease on initial diagnosis by 40% and 75%, respectively [5,6].

Commonly accepted risk factors for PCa include age, African race, several genetic factors and a family history of PCa [7]. More specifically, PCa is considered to be one of the malignancies with the greatest heritability component (up to 57% genetic contribution) [8], with several studies suggesting that 8–12% of all patients presenting with advanced disease may harbor a germline mutation in a tumor-suppressor gene [9,10]. Interestingly, it has been shown that individuals with a family history of PCa have 2.5 times higher probability of being diagnosed with the same disease when compared to the general population [11]. Researchers analyzing data form the Swedish Cancer Database concluded that the three malignancies with the highest familial cancer rate are prostate, breast and colorectal cancer (20.2% vs. 13.6% vs. 12.8%) [12]. An integrative analysis on patients diagnosed with advanced disease showed that somatic and germline alterations were found in up to 90% of those suffering from metastatic castration-resistant cancer [13]. So far, the most well-studied germline mutations relating to PCa are those of BRCA 1/2, CHEK2, NBM and ATM [10,14,15].

The main scope of the current review is to specifically examine the impact of BRCA mutations in the context of PCa, as well as their significance as a genetic biomarker in the era of efforts towards personalized screening. Emphasis is given to studies discussing prostate cancer risk stratification and early prostate cancer detection. Since our aim was to perform a narrative review, we included only "landmark" publications.

2. Role of Family History and BRCA Genes in PCa

In 2015, a study conducted by Liss et al. showed that male patients who had a history of PCa in their families were not only more susceptible to developing the same malignancy but they were also at a greater risk of dying from PCa, with both results being statistically significant. The same study highlighted the value of early PSA testing in family members of PCa patients, as it can lead to lower cancer-specific mortality rates and a possible survival benefit [16]. Likewise, a study performed by Brandt et al. showed that the hazard ratios for prostate cancer diagnosis and risk of death from prostate cancer in men increased with the number of affected relatives and decreased with increased age [17]. Also worth noting is the fact that we should treat familial and hereditary cancer as two distinct clinical entities. The hereditary form can be attributed to identifiable mutations (most commonly mutations regarding BRCA genes), while the familial form covers a larger spectrum (approximately 15–20% of PCa cases), with individuals having a positive family history in common but no identifiable genetic alteration. Nevertheless, the degree to which a positive family history defines the probability of developing cancer is highly variable and is also affected by factors such as age and degree of relation with the affected individuals. According to Carter et al., the proportion of PCa cases that could be attributed to mutated high-risk alleles was found to be approximately equal to 40% for men younger than 55 years, which is much higher than the 9% for individuals older than 85 years [18]. Moreover, a meta-analysis conducted by Zeeger et al. showed that men with an affected father had more than 50% lower relative risk of receiving a diagnosis of PCa than men with an affected brother (2.2 vs. 3.4), whereas this risk practically disappeared among second-degree family members [19]. Bratt et al. provided a nationwide population study, reporting the association between family history and diagnosis of prostate cancer in different cancer risk categories (any prostate cancer, non-low-risk prostate cancer and high-risk prostate cancer). According to them, the probabilities of intermediate and high-risk prostate cancer are better for counselling men with a positive family history of prostate cancer [20]. Having this in mind, it is easy to understand that in order to achieve a better estimation of the lifetime risk of being diagnosed with PCa, based solely on heritability factors, we should take into consideration the status of close relatives as well as the number of affected individuals in a family pedigree and their age at diagnosis. In this diagnostic algorithm, we should also take into account a family history from the maternal family branch [21].

BRCA 1 and BRCA 2 genes were first discovered almost three decades ago (1994 and 1995, respectively) after carefully examining the biological and genetic background of families with an abnormally high prevalence of breast and ovarian cancer [22,23]. These genes are responsible for 30–70% and approximately 90% of all hereditary breast and ovarian cancer cases, respectively. According to several studies, individuals harboring mutations in these genes have a lifetime risk of developing breast cancer of up to 85%, while the risk for ovarian cancer ranges from 20 to 40%. Individuals carrying BRCA1 mutations were also found to be at higher risk of developing other types of cancer, such as pancreatic and cervical. As far as prostate cancer is concerned, the risk was found to be age-dependent, affecting carriers younger than 65 years old [24,25].

In terms of biology, BRCA genes belong to the family of DNA damage repair (DDR) genes. The main role of these genes is to repair several DNA aberrations taking place during the cell cycle, thus providing genomic stability and ensuring an uneventful distribution of genetic material to the daughter cells following mitotic cell division [26]. In cases where this system fails, individuals become susceptible to malignancies such as breast, ovarian, prostate and pancreatic cancer. In particular, BRCA 1 mutations were associated with an increased risk of ovarian and breast cancer, whereas BRCA 2 carriers were more susceptible to pancreatic and prostate cancer [27]. According to several studies, the percentage of patients with PCa that harbor a BRCA2 mutation ranges between 1.2% and 3.2%, and the percentage is even smaller when it comes to BRCA1 [28,29]. Nevertheless, those genes (especially BRCA2) are considered to be responsible for most cases of hereditary PCa, with mutations in BRCA2 and BRCA1 increasing the risk by 3–8.6 times and up to 4 times, respectively, when compared to the general population [24,28,30,31].

So far, several studies have shown that PCa in individuals with mutated BRCA1/2 genes is in general more aggressive and associated with lower overall survival when compared to cases of male patients with normal alleles [32–35]. Back in 2019, Castro et al. conducted a retrospective analysis based on data from 79 BRCA mutation carriers and 1940 non-carriers, all of whom were diagnosed with PCa [33]. According to the authors, BRCA 1/2 mutations were found to be directly correlated with a higher risk of locally advanced disease, a higher Gleason score, nodal infiltration and distant metastases at the time of diagnosis. Moreover, they showed that BRCA2 mutations should be considered an independent negative prognostic factor based on both the significantly shorter 5-year cancer-specific survival and metastasis-free survival among mutation carriers.

Just to further examine the strength of the connection between BRCA mutations and PCa risk, Ibrahim et al. carried out a retrospective analysis by dividing a total of 102 men into two cohorts based on their genetic profile (mutation of either BRCA1 or BRCA2) [36]. Based on their findings, almost one-third of the under-examination individuals had at least one type of cancer, with prostate cancer being the most common (2 patients in the BRCA1 group and 11 patients in the BRCA2 group), followed by breast, skin and urothelial cancer. The above findings are in accordance with previous studies, supporting the theory that BRCA2 mutation carriers are far more susceptible to malignancies than BRCA1 carriers [25,30,37–39]. According to a well-designed case–control study on a special population of males of Ashkenazi origin, BRCA2 mutation carriers were shown to be at greater risk of developing PCa when compared to the age-matched control group [40]. Finally, according to the PROREPAIR-B trial, which prospectively examined only patients with metastatic castration-resistant disease, a germline BRCA2 mutation was characterized as an independent negative prognostic factor with a statistically significant lower CSS rate (17.4 vs. 33.2 months, $p = 0.027$). In this particular study, a statistically significant difference was also noticed in terms of treating BRCA2 carriers; namely, the use of ARTA (abiraterone or enzalutamide) was associated with better CSS and PFS in comparison with taxanes [41].

3. BRCA Testing in Prostate Cancer and Screening of Men with Known Mutations

Nowadays, it has become clear that PSA, which has been established as the major screening tool for PCa detection, has contributed to a small absolute decrease regarding the risk of death from PCa [42], while bringing with it the risk of overdiagnosis and the unnecessary treatment of quite a few individuals who would otherwise have never experienced clinical manifestations of the disease [43]. Under these circumstances, we can easily understand that a universal screening plan is related to a high financial burden as well as several unnecessary biopsies and treatment-related morbidities for individuals with indolent disease and a high PSA value [44,45]. On the other hand, we cannot overlook the importance of disease detection at an earlier stage, which gives us the opportunity to use a variety of therapeutic interventions with the aim of preventing cancer progression and metastatic disease [46]. Having all the above in mind, it is easy to justify the efforts made in recent years towards finding sufficient and objective data that could support the development of individualized screening plans. In the process of planning such strategies, we should take into consideration not only results from recent studies and population stratification tactics but also the need for shared and informed decision making.

In general, when we suspect the presence of an inherited malignancy or syndrome running through a family, it is of utmost importance that the patient is referred for genetic counseling. Unfortunately, in the case of PCa, there has been no uniform consensus so far regarding the exact criteria that should lead a patient to visit a geneticist.

In the context of PCa, without specific consideration of any particular genetic alteration, the American College of Medical Genetics suggests that a thorough genetic evaluation should take place if any of the following stands true [47]:

1. Two or more relatives receiving a PCa diagnosis at an age of 55 or younger (the relatives should be first-degree).
2. At least three first-degree relatives with PCa, irrespective of age.
3. Gleason grade 8 or higher and at least two individuals in the family pedigree diagnosed with breast, ovarian or pancreatic cancer.

Again, without specific interest for a specific mutation, the Johns Hopkins groups suggests another set of guidelines for familial PCa, which are as follows [48]:

1. Family pedigree with evidence of PCa in three successive generations.
2. Two relatives diagnosed with PCa at an early age ($\leq$55 years).
3. At least three first-degree relatives with PCa.

Based on EAU recommendations, all individuals with high-risk or metastatic disease should be offered genetic counseling at least for the possibility that they have mutations in the BRCA1/2, ATM, FANCA or PALB2 genes. For the patients who are diagnosed with lower-risk disease, testing is recommended if any of the following are true [49]:

1. There is a strong family history of PCa.
2. At least one member of the family is diagnosed with Lynch syndrome.
3. There are already known germline mutations in the family or at least one family member has pancreatic or breast or ovarian cancer (possible BRCA2 mutation).

On the other hand, the National Comprehensive Cancer Network (NCCN) has published guidelines specifically for testing BRCA1/BRCA2 status, including patients with any of the following characteristics [50]:

1. Diagnosis of PCa (Gleason $\geq$ 7) and at least two relatives with prostate (Gleason $\geq$ 7) or breast or pancreatic cancer.
2. Metastatic PCa (proven with biopsy or imaging test).
3. Diagnosis of PCa (Gleason $\geq$ 7) at any age and at least one close relative with breast (age $\leq$ 50 years) or invasive ovarian cancer.

Serious efforts to reach a consensus and possibly bridge the gap between the recommendations made by different organizations have been made through studies like IMPACT. This study is an ongoing multicenter observational trial on carriers of BRCA1/2 mutations who have already been diagnosed with PCa [51]. The main purpose of the study is to determine the significance of an annual PSA testing protocol for BRCA1/2 carriers compared with non-carriers, with the PSA threshold for a biopsy being that of 3 ng/mL. In their interim analysis, researchers concluded that further follow-up is needed for BRCA1 carriers, but as regards the BRCA2 carriers, early and routine screening with PSA is important, as it was demonstrated that prostate biopsy in this specific population is associated with twice the positive predictive value compared to general population studies. An interim analysis of the IMPACT study showed that 77% of BRCA2 carriers were diagnosed with intermediate and high-risk disease [52]. A Dutch multidisciplinary expert panel reached a consensus in a meeting regarding the indications and applications of germline and tumor genetic testing in prostate cancer. Interestingly, they agreed that germline and tumor genetic testing should not be performed in the case of nonmetastatic hormone-sensitive prostate cancer when a relevant family history of cancer does not exist. As far as the metastatic disease is concerned, neither of the above-mentioned tests received panel approval for implementation in M1a HSPC, whereas it was agreed that the final therapeutic decision was not affected by the results. In metastatic CRPC, there was a lack of consensus regarding when tumor genetic testing should be performed and who should evaluate it, thus coming to no recommendations [53]. Table 1 summarizes the recommendations of different organizations for genetic testing in prostate cancer.

Table 1. Genetic testing recommendations for prostate cancer according to different organizations.

Organization	Gene Testing	Patient Characteristics
American College of Medical Genetics.	Thorough genetic evaluation.	1. Two or more first-degree relatives receiving a PCa diagnosis at an age of 55 or younger. 2. At least three first-degree relatives with PCa, irrespective of age. 3. Gleason grade 8 or higher and at least two individuals in the family pedigree diagnosed with breast, ovarian or pancreatic cancer.
Johns Hopkins groups.	Thorough genetic evaluation.	1. Family pedigree with evidence of PCa in three successive generations. 2. Two relatives diagnosed with PCa at an age of 55 or younger. 3. At least three first-degree relatives with PCa.
European Association of Urology (EAU) Recommendations.	Genetic counseling at least for the possibility that they have mutations in BRCA1/2, ATM, FANCA or PALB2 genes.	All individuals with high-risk or metastatic disease. For the patients who are diagnosed with lower-risk disease, testing is recommended if [49]: 1. There is a strong family history of PCa. 2. At least one member of the family is diagnosed with Lynch syndrome. 3. There are already known germline mutations in the family or at least one family member has pancreatic or breast or ovarian cancer (possible BRCA2 mutation).
National Comprehensive Cancer Network (NCCN).	Specific BRCA1/BRCA2 status.	1. Diagnosis of PCa (Gleason $\geq$ 7) and at least two relatives with prostate (Gleason $\geq$ 7) or breast or pancreatic cancer. 2. Metastatic PCa (proven with biopsy or imaging test). 3. Diagnosis of PCa (Gleason $\geq$ 7) at any age and at least one close relative with breast (age $\leq$ 50 years) or invasive ovarian cancer.

In an effort to establish risk-adapted guidelines for PCa diagnosis, the NCCN recommends that BRCA1/2 carriers should be tested annually starting at the age of 40 years [54]. The EAU follows the same directions with the exceptions of recommending intervals based upon the baseline PSA value and not including BRCA1 carriers in their guidelines [55]. Finally, the ACS does not take into consideration the germline status and suggests that men with a first-degree relative diagnosed younger than 65 years should start screening at 40 years (45 years if more than one first-degree relative with PCa) [56]. A recent review article by Giri et al. summarizes all existing guidelines for germline testing in prostate cancer, in an effort to promote multidisciplinary patient primary care. The authors also shed light on a very intriguing topic, namely the involvement of primary care physicians in the genetic testing process and algorithm. Through proper education, these professionals can offer individualized patient-centered medical advice and refer individuals with a positive family history at high risk for further evaluation and assessment by specialists [57].

4. Conclusions

Genetic studies during recent decades have undoubtedly added a lot to our current understanding of prostate cancer biology. Based on the current literature, it seems to be inevitable that genetic testing is very soon going to be an integral part of clinical practice not only for individuals already diagnosed with the disease but also in the setting of population screening. Hopefully, more precise knowledge on genetic predispositions for PCa is going to help us further improve our risk assessment strategies and achieve better results for our patients and their families.

Author Contributions: Conceptualization, N.G., N.K., D.M. and H.v.d.P.; methodology, T.S., N.K., C.Z., M.K., I.L. and I.K.; formal analysis, N.K., T.S. and C.Z.; writing—original draft preparation, T.S., N.K. and N.G.; writing—review and editing, T.S., D.M., C.Z, N.K., I.L., M.K., I.K. and H.v.d.P.; supervision, H.v.d.P. and D.M. All authors have read and agreed to the published version of the manuscript.

Funding: This research received no external funding.

Data Availability Statement: No new data were created.

Conflicts of Interest: The authors declare no conflicts of interest.

References

1. Torre, L.A.; Bray, F.; Siegel, R.L.; Ferlay, J.; Lortet-Tieulent, J.; Jemal, A. Global cancer statistics, 2012. *CA Cancer J. Clin.* **2015**, *65*, 87–108. [CrossRef] [PubMed]
2. Siegel, R.L.; Miller, K.D.; Jemal, A. Cancer statistics, 2020. *CA Cancer J. Clin.* **2020**, *70*, 7–30. [CrossRef] [PubMed]
3. National Cancer Institute SEER Cancer Statistics Factsheets. Prostate Cancer. 2020. Available online: https://seer.cancer.gov/statfacts/html/prost.html (accessed on 4 September 2020).
4. Lin, D.W.; Porter, M.; Montgomery, B. Treatment and survival outcomes in young men diagnosed with prostate cancer: A Population-based Cohort Study. *Cancer* **2009**, *115*, 2863–2871. [CrossRef] [PubMed]
5. Kohler, B.A.; Ward, E.; McCarthy, B.J.; Schymura, M.J.; Ries, L.A.; Eheman, C.; Jemal, A.; Anderson, R.N.; Ajani, U.A.; Edwards, B.K. Annual report to the nation on the status of cancer, 1975–2007, featuring tumors of the brain and other nervous system. *J. Natl. Cancer Inst.* **2011**, *103*, 714–736. [CrossRef] [PubMed]
6. Scosyrev, E.; Wu, G.; Mohile, S.; Messing, E.M. Prostate-specific antigen screening for prostate cancer and the risk of overt metastatic disease at presentation: Analysis of trends over time. *Cancer* **2012**, *118*, 5768–5776. [CrossRef] [PubMed]
7. Pernar, C.H.; Ebot, E.M.; Wilson, K.M.; Mucci, L.A. The Epidemiology of Prostate Cancer. *Cold Spring Harb. Perspect. Med.* **2018**, *8*, a030361. [CrossRef]
8. Mucci, L.A.; Hjelmborg, J.B.; Harris, J.R.; Czene, K.; Havelick, D.J.; Scheike, T.; Graff, R.E.; Holst, K.; Möller, S.; Unger, R.H.; et al. Nordic Twin Study of Cancer (NorTwinCan) Collaboration. Familial Risk and Heritability of Cancer Among Twins in Nordic Countries. *JAMA* **2016**, *315*, 68–76, Erratum in *JAMA* **2016**, *315*, 822. [CrossRef]
9. Leongamornlert, D.; Saunders, E.; Dadaev, T.; Tymrakiewicz, M.; Goh, C.; Jugurnauth-Little, S.; Kozarewa, I.; Fenwick, K.; Assiotis, I.; Barrowdale, D.; et al. Frequent germline deleterious mutations in DNA repair genes in familial prostate cancer cases are associated with advanced disease. *Br. J. Cancer* **2014**, *110*, 1663–1672. [CrossRef]
10. Pritchard, C.C.; Mateo, J.; Walsh, M.F.; De Sarkar, N.; Abida, W.; Beltran, H.; Garofalo, A.; Gulati, R.; Carreira, S.; Eeles, R.; et al. Inherited DNA-Repair Gene Mutations in Men with Metastatic Prostate Cancer. *N. Engl. J. Med.* **2016**, *375*, 443–453. [CrossRef]
11. Johns, L.E.; Houlston, R.S. A systematic review and meta-analysis of familial prostate cancer risk. *BJU Int.* **2003**, *91*, 789–794. [CrossRef]
12. Verhage, B.A.; Aben, K.K.; Witjes, J.A.; Straatman, H.; Schalken, J.A.; Kiemeney, L.A. Site-specific familial aggregation of prostate cancer. *Int. J. Cancer* **2004**, *109*, 611–617. [CrossRef]
13. Robinson, D.; Van Allen, E.M.; Wu, Y.M.; Schultz, N.; Lonigro, R.J.; Mosquera, J.M.; Montgomery, B.; Taplin, M.E.; Pritchard, C.C.; Attard, G.; et al. Integrative clinical genomics of advanced prostate cancer. *Cell* **2015**, *161*, 1215–1228, Erratum in *Cell* **2015**, *162*, 454. [CrossRef]
14. Na, R.; Zheng, S.L.; Han, M.; Yu, H.; Jiang, D.; Shah, S.; Ewing, C.M.; Zhang, L.; Novakovic, K.; Petkewicz, J.; et al. Germline Mutations in ATM and BRCA1/2 Distinguish Risk for Lethal and Indolent Prostate Cancer and are Associated with Early Age at Death. *Eur. Urol.* **2017**, *71*, 740–747. [CrossRef] [PubMed]
15. Giri, V.N.; Knudsen, K.E.; Kelly, W.K.; Cheng, H.H.; Cooney, K.A.; Cookson, M.S.; Dahut, W.; Weissman, S.; Soule, H.R.; Petrylak, D.P.; et al. Implementation of Germline Testing for Prostate Cancer: Philadelphia Prostate Cancer Consensus Conference 2019. *J. Clin. Oncol.* **2020**, *38*, 2798–2811. [CrossRef]
16. Liss, M.A.; Chen, H.; Hemal, S.; Krane, S.; Kane, C.J.; Xu, J.; Kader, A.K. Impact of family history on prostate cancer mortality in white men undergoing prostate specific antigen based screening. *J. Urol.* **2015**, *193*, 75–79. [CrossRef]
17. Brandt, A.; Bermejo, J.L.; Sundquist, J.; Hemminki, K. Age-specific risk of incident prostate cancer and risk of death from prostate cancer defined by the number of affected family members. *Eur. Urol.* **2010**, *58*, 275–280. [CrossRef] [PubMed]
18. Carter, B.S.; Bova, G.S.; Beaty, T.H.; Steinberg, G.D.; Childs, B.; Isaacs, W.B.; Walsh, P.C. Hereditary prostate cancer: Epidemiologic and clinical features. *J. Urol.* **1993**, *150*, 797–802. [CrossRef] [PubMed]
19. Zeegers, M.P.; Jellema, A.; Ostrer, H. Empiric risk of prostate carcinoma for relatives of patients with prostate carcinoma: A meta-analysis. *Cancer* **2003**, *97*, 1894–1903. [CrossRef] [PubMed]

20. Bratt, O.; Drevin, L.; Akre, O.; Garmo, H.; Stattin, P. Family History and Probability of Prostate Cancer, Differentiated by Risk Category: A Nationwide Population-Based Study. *J. Natl. Cancer Inst.* **2016**, *108*, djw110. [CrossRef]
21. Albright, F.; Stephenson, R.A.; Agarwal, N.; Teerlink, C.C.; Lowrance, W.T.; Farnham, J.M.; Albright, L.A. Prostate cancer risk prediction based on complete prostate cancer family history. *Prostate* **2015**, *75*, 390–398. [CrossRef]
22. Miki, Y.; Swensen, J.; Shattuck-Eidens, D.; Futreal, P.A.; Harshman, K.; Tavtigian, S.; Liu, Q.; Cochran, C.; Bennett, L.M.; Ding, W.; et al. A strong candidate for the breast and ovarian cancer susceptibility gene BRCA1. *Science* **1994**, *266*, 66–71. [CrossRef]
23. Wooster, R.; Bignell, G.; Lancaster, J.; Swift, S.; Seal, S.; Mangion, J.; Collins, N.; Gregory, S.; Gumbs, C.; Micklem, G. Identification of the breast cancer susceptibility gene BRCA2. *Nature* **1995**, *378*, 789–892, Erratum in *Nature* **1996**, *379*, 749. [CrossRef]
24. Thompson, D.; Easton, D.F.; Breast Cancer Linkage Consortium. Cancer Incidence in BRCA1 mutation carriers. *J. Natl. Cancer Inst.* **2002**, *94*, 1358–1365. [CrossRef]
25. Breast Cancer Linkage Consortium. Cancer risks in BRCA2 mutation carriers. *J. Natl. Cancer Inst.* **1999**, *91*, 1310–1316. [CrossRef]
26. Reinhardt, H.C.; Yaffe, M.B. Phospho-Ser/Thr-binding domains: Navigating the cell cycle and DNA damage response. *Nat. Rev. Mol. Cell Biol.* **2013**, *14*, 563–580. [CrossRef]
27. Mersch, J.; Jackson, M.A.; Park, M.; Nebgen, D.; Peterson, S.K.; Singletary, C.; Arun, B.K.; Litton, J.K. Cancers associated with BRCA1 and BRCA2 mutations other than breast and ovarian. *Cancer* **2015**, *121*, 269–275, Erratum in *Cancer* **2015**, *121*, 2474–2475. [CrossRef] [PubMed]
28. Gallagher, D.J.; Gaudet, M.M.; Pal, P.; Kirchhoff, T.; Balistreri, L.; Vora, K.; Bhatia, J.; Stadler, Z.; Fine, S.W.; Reuter, V.; et al. Germline BRCA mutations denote a clinicopathologic subset of prostate cancer. *Clin. Cancer Res.* **2010**, *16*, 2115–2121. [CrossRef] [PubMed]
29. Giusti, R.M.; Rutter, J.L.; Duray, P.H.; Freedman, L.S.; Konichezky, M.; Fisher-Fischbein, J.; Greene, M.H.; Maslansky, B.; Fischbein, A.; Gruber, S.B.; et al. A twofold increase in BRCA mutation related prostate cancer among Ashkenazi Israelis is not associated with distinctive histopathology. *J. Med. Genet.* **2003**, *40*, 787–792, Erratum in *J. Med. Genet.* **2004**, *41*, 51. [CrossRef]
30. Kote-Jarai, Z.; Leongamornlert, D.; Saunders, E.; Tymrakiewicz, M.; Castro, E.; Mahmud, N.; Guy, M.; Edwards, S.; O'Brien, L.; Sawyer, E.; et al. BRCA2 is a moderate penetrance gene contributing to young-onset prostate cancer: Implications for genetic testing in prostate cancer patients. *Br. J. Cancer* **2011**, *105*, 1230–1234. [CrossRef] [PubMed]
31. Venkitaraman, A.R. Cancer susceptibility and the functions of BRCA1 and BRCA2. *Cell* **2002**, *108*, 171–182. [CrossRef]
32. Mitra, A.V.; Bancroft, E.K.; Barbachano, Y.; Page, E.C.; Foster, C.S.; Jameson, C.; Mitchell, G.; Lindeman, G.J.; Stapleton, A.; Suthers, G.; et al. Targeted prostate cancer screening in men with mutations in BRCA1 and BRCA2 detects aggressive prostate cancer: Preliminary analysis of the results of the IMPACT study. *BJU Int.* **2011**, *107*, 28–39. [CrossRef] [PubMed]
33. Castro, E.; Goh, C.; Olmos, D.; Saunders, E.; Leongamornlert, D.; Tymrakiewicz, M.; Mahmud, N.; Dadaev, T.; Govindasami, K.; Guy, M.; et al. Germline BRCA mutations are associated with higher risk of nodal involvement, distant metastasis, and poor survival outcomes in prostate cancer. *J. Clin. Oncol.* **2013**, *31*, 1748–1757. [CrossRef]
34. Mitra, A.; Fisher, C.; Foster, C.S.; Jameson, C.; Barbachanno, Y.; Bartlett, J.; Bancroft, E.; Doherty, R.; Kote-Jarai, Z.; Peock, S.; et al. Prostate cancer in male BRCA1 and BRCA2 mutation carriers has a more aggressive phenotype. *Br. J. Cancer* **2008**, *98*, 502–507. [CrossRef] [PubMed]
35. Thorne, H.; Willems, A.J.; Niedermayr, E.; Hoh, I.M.; Li, J.; Clouston, D.; Mitchell, G.; Fox, S.; Hopper, J.L.; Kathleen Cunningham Consortium for Research in Familial Breast Cancer Consortium; et al. Decreased prostate cancer-specific survival of men with BRCA2 mutations from multiple breast cancer families. *Cancer Prev. Res. (Phila)* **2011**, *4*, 1002–1010. [CrossRef] [PubMed]
36. Ibrahim, M.; Yadav, S.; Ogunleye, F.; Zakalik, D. Male BRCA mutation carriers: Clinical characteristics and cancer spectrum. *BMC Cancer* **2018**, *18*, 179. [CrossRef]
37. Tai, Y.C.; Domchek, S.; Parmigiani, G.; Chen, S. Breast cancer risk among male BRCA1 and BRCA2 mutation carriers. *J. Natl. Cancer Inst.* **2007**, *99*, 1811–1814. [CrossRef]
38. Evans, D.G.; Susnerwala, I.; Dawson, J.; Woodward, E.; Maher, E.R.; Lalloo, F. Risk of breast cancer in male BRCA2 carriers. *J. Med. Genet.* **2010**, *47*, 710–711. [CrossRef]
39. Moran, A.; O'Hara, C.; Khan, S.; Shack, L.; Woodward, E.; Maher, E.R.; Lalloo, F.; Evans, D.G. Risk of cancer other than breast or ovarian in individuals with BRCA1 and BRCA2 mutations. *Fam. Cancer* **2012**, *11*, 235–242. [CrossRef]
40. Kirchhoff, T.; Kauff, N.D.; Mitra, N.; Nafa, K.; Huang, H.; Palmer, C.; Gulati, T.; Wadsworth, E.; Donat, S.; Robson, M.E.; et al. BRCA mutations and risk of prostate cancer in Ashkenazi Jews. *Clin. Cancer Res.* **2004**, *10*, 2918–2921. [CrossRef]
41. Castro, E.; Romero-Laorden, N.; Del Pozo, A.; Lozano, R.; Medina, A.; Puente, J.; Piulats, J.M.; Lorente, D.; Saez, M.I.; Morales-Barrera, R.; et al. PROREPAIR-B: A Prospective Cohort Study of the Impact of Germline DNA Repair Mutations on the Outcomes of Patients With Metastatic Castration-Resistant Prostate Cancer. *J. Clin. Oncol.* **2019**, *37*, 490–503. [CrossRef]
42. Schröder, F.H.; Hugosson, J.; Roobol, M.J.; Tammela, T.L.; Ciatto, S.; Nelen, V.; Kwiatkowski, M.; Lujan, M.; Lilja, H.; Zappa, M.; et al. Screening and prostate-cancer mortality in a randomized European study. *N. Engl. J. Med.* **2009**, *360*, 1320–1328. [CrossRef]
43. Ilic, D.; Neuberger, M.M.; Djulbegovic, M.; Dahm, P. Screening for prostate cancer. *Cochrane Database Syst. Rev.* **2013**, *2013*, CD004720. [CrossRef]
44. US Preventive Services Task Force; Grossman, D.C.; Curry, S.J.; Owens, D.K.; Bibbins-Domingo, K.; Caughey, A.B.; Davidson, K.W.; Doubeni, C.A.; Ebell, M.; Epling, J.W., Jr.; et al. Screening for Prostate Cancer: US Preventive Services Task Force Recommendation Statement. *JAMA* **2018**, *319*, 1901–1913, Erratum in *JAMA* **2018**, *319*, 2443. [CrossRef] [PubMed]

45. Wolf, A.M.; Wender, R.C.; Etzioni, R.B.; Thompson, I.M.; D'Amico, A.V.; Volk, R.J.; Brooks, D.D.; Dash, C.; Guessous, I.; Andrews, K.; et al. American Cancer Society guideline for the early detection of prostate cancer: Update 2010. *CA Cancer J Clin.* **2010**, *60*, 70–98. [CrossRef]
46. Hamdy, F.C.; Donovan, J.L.; Lane, J.A.; Mason, M.; Metcalfe, C.; Holding, P.; Davis, M.; Peters, T.J.; Turner, E.L.; Martin, R.M.; et al. 10-Year Outcomes after Monitoring, Surgery, or Radiotherapy for Localized Prostate Cancer. *N. Engl. J. Med.* **2016**, *375*, 1415–1424. [CrossRef] [PubMed]
47. Hampel, H.; Bennett, R.L.; Buchanan, A.; Pearlman, R.; Wiesner, G.L.; Guideline Development Group, American College of Medical Genetics and Genomics Professional Practice and Guidelines Committee and National Society of Genetic Counselors Practice Guidelines Committee. A practice guideline from the American College of Medical Genetics and Genomics and the National Society of Genetic Counselors: Referral indications for cancer predisposition assessment. *Genet. Med.* **2015**, *17*, 70–87. [CrossRef] [PubMed]
48. Bova, G.S.; Partin, A.W.; Isaacs, S.D.; Carter, B.S.; Beaty, T.L.; Isaacs, W.B.; Walsh, P.C. Biological aggressiveness of hereditary prostate cancer: Long-term evaluation following radical prostatectomy. *J. Urol.* **1998**, *160 Pt 1*, 660–663. [CrossRef]
49. Heidegger, I.; Tsaur, I.; Borgmann, H.; Surcel, C.; Kretschmer, A.; Mathieu, R.; Visschere, P.; Valerio, M.; van den Bergh, R.C.N.; Ost, P.; et al. Hereditary prostate cancer—Primetime for genetic testing? *Cancer Treat. Rev.* **2019**, *81*, 101927. [CrossRef] [PubMed]
50. National Comprehensive Cancer Network (NCCN). *Genetic/Familial High-Risk Assessment: Breast and Ovarian (Version 1.2018)*; NCCN: Fort Washington, PA, USA, 2018.
51. Bancroft, E.K.; Page, E.C.; Castro, E.; Lilja, H.; Vickers, A.; Sjoberg, D.; Assel, M.; Foster, C.S.; Mitchell, G.; Drew, K.; et al. Targeted prostate cancer screening in BRCA1 and BRCA2 mutation carriers: Results from the initial screening round of the IMPACT study. *Eur. Urol.* **2014**, *66*, 489–499, Erratum in *Eur. Urol.* **2015**, *67*, e126. [CrossRef]
52. Page, E.C.; Bancroft, E.K.; Brook, M.N.; Assel, M.; Hassan Al Battat, M.; Thomas, S.; Taylor, N.; Chamberlain, A.; Pope, J.; Raghallaigh, H.N.; et al. Interim Results from the IMPACT Study: Evidence for Prostate-specific Antigen Screening in BRCA2 Mutation Carriers. *Eur. Urol.* **2019**, *76*, 831–842. [CrossRef]
53. Mehra, N.; Kloots, I.; Vlaming, M.; Aluwini, S.; Dewulf, E.; Oprea-Lager, D.E.; van der Poel, H.; Stoevelaar, H.; Yakar, D.; Bangma, C.H.; et al. Genetic Aspects and Molecular Testing in Prostate Cancer: A Report from a Dutch Multidisciplinary Consensus Meeting. *Eur. Urol. Open Sci.* **2023**, *49*, 23–31. [CrossRef] [PubMed]
54. National Comprehensive Cancer Network. *NCCN Clinical Practice Guidelines in Oncology: Prostate Cancer Early Dectection*; National Comprehensive Cancer Network: Plymouth Meeting, PA, USA, 2020; Available online: https://www.nccn.org/professionals/physician_gls/pdf/prostate_detection.pdf (accessed on 15 October 2020).
55. Mottet, N.; Cornford, P.; van den Bergh, R.C.N.; Briers, E.; De Santis, M.; Fanti, S. Prostate cancer. In *EAU Guidelines*; European Association of Urology, Ed.; European Association of Urology: Arnhem, The Netherlands, 2020; pp. 1–212.
56. American Cancer Society. *Cancer A-Z: Prostate Cancer Early Detection, Diagnosis, and Staging*; American Cancer Society: Atlanta, GA, USA, 2019; Available online: https://www.cancer.org/content/dam/CRC/PDF/Public/8795.00.pdf (accessed on 16 October 2023).
57. Giri, V.N.; Morgan, T.M.; Morris, D.S.; Berchuck, J.E.; Hyatt, C.; Taplin, M.E. Genetic testing in prostate cancer management: Considerations informing primary care. *CA Cancer J. Clin.* **2022**, *72*, 360–371. [CrossRef] [PubMed]

Current Oncology

MDPI

Article

MRI-Targeted Prostate Fusion Biopsy: What Are We Missing outside the Target? Implications for Treatment Planning

Marco Oderda [1,*], Alessandro Dematteis [1], Giorgio Calleris [1], Romain Diamand [2], Marco Gatti [3], Giancarlo Marra [1], Gilles Adans-Dester [4], Yazan Al Salhi [5], Antonio Pastore [5], Riccardo Faletti [3] and Paolo Gontero [1]

1 Division of Urology, Department of Surgical Sciences, Molinette Hospital, University of Turin, 10126 Torino, Italy; dmtlsn@gmail.com (A.D.); giorgio.calleris@unito.it (G.C.); giancarlo.marra@unito.it (G.M.); paolo.gontero@unito.it (P.G.)
2 Department of Urology, Jules Bordet Institute—Erasme Hospital, Hôpital Universitaire de Bruxelles, Université Libre de Bruxelles, 1070 Brussels, Belgium; romain.diamand@ulb.be
3 Division of Radiology, Department of Surgical Sciences, Molinette Hospital, University of Turin, 10126 Torino, Italy; marco.gatti@unito.it (M.G.); riccardo.faletti@unito.it (R.F.)
4 Department of Urology, Centre Hospitalier Universitaire Namur-Godinne, UCLouvain, 5530 Yvoir, Belgium; gilles.adans-dester@chuuclnamur.uclouvain.be
5 Urology Unit, Department of Medico-Surgical Sciences and Biotechnologies, Sapienza University of Rome, 04100 Latina, Italy; yazan.alsalhi@uniroma1.it (Y.A.S.); antonioluigi.pastore@uniroma1.it (A.P.)
* Correspondence: marco.oderda@unito.it; Tel.: +39-3479383465

Abstract: Introduction: This study aimed to evaluate the added diagnostic value of systematic biopsies (SBx) after magnetic resonance imaging (MRI)-targeted biopsies (TBx) and the presence of prostate cancer (PCa) outside MRI targets, in a prospective, contemporary, multicentric series of fusion biopsy patients. **Methods**: We collected data on 962 consecutive patients who underwent fusion biopsy between 2022 and 2024. Prostate cancer was considered clinically significant (csPCa) in the case of grade ≥ 2. Median test and Fisher exact chi-square tests were used. To identify predictors of out-field positivity, univariate and multivariable logistic regression analyses were performed. **Results**: Prostate cancer and csPCa were detected by TBx only in 56% and 50%, respectively, and by SBx only in 55% and 45%, respectively ($p < 0.001$). Prostate cancer and csPCa were diagnosed by TBx in 100 (10%) and 82 (8%) SBx-negative cases and by SBx in 86 (9%) and 54 (6%) TBx-negative cases ($p < 0.001$). Tumors outside MRI targets were found in 213 (33%) cases in the same lobe and 208 (32%) in the contralateral lobe, most of them being csPCa. Predictors of out-field contralateral PCa were positive DRE (HR 1.50, p 0.03), PSA density ≥ 0.15 (HR 2.20, $p < 0.001$), and PI-RADS score 5 (HR 2.04, p 0.01). **Conclusions**: Both TBx and SBx identify a non-negligible proportion of csPCa when the other modality is negative. SBx after TBx should always be considered given the risk of missing other csPCa foci within the prostate, especially in patients with positive DRE, PSA density ≥ 0.15, and PIRADS 5 lesions.

Keywords: prostate biopsy; fusion; out-field; outside; MRI; accuracy

1. Introduction

Multiparametric magnetic resonance imaging (MRI) is essential in the diagnosis of prostate cancer (PCa) and is recommended in patients with clinical suspicion of PCa. If a suspicious lesion is found on MRI, MRI-targeted prostate biopsy (TBx) is advised, together with a systematic mapping [1]. The need for systematic biopsies (SBxs) is supported by a risk of missing approximately 16% and 10% of clinically significant PCa (csPCa) in biopsy-naïve and repeat-biopsy patients, according to a recent Cochrane meta-analysis [2]. However, the performance of supplementary mapping is increasingly being questioned, considering that several studies demonstrated a limited added diagnostic benefit of 5% to 7% [3,4]. A recent multicentric study that evaluated the added value in csPCa detection of side-specific SBx relative to an MRI lesion found that biopsies taken at the opposite side of the MRI-suspicious lesion have only a negligible impact on per-patient cancer detection [5]. Nevertheless, SBx has been suggested to detect a high number of PCa foci outside mpMRI targets, improving the assessment of the tumor burden inside the prostate [6]. Considering the multifocal nature of PCa, a thorough knowledge of the location of all cancer foci inside the prostate is essential for a correct treatment decision. In the present study, we evaluated the added diagnostic value of SBx and the presence of PCa outside MRI targets, in a prospective, contemporary, multicentric series of fusion biopsy patients.

2. Patients and Methods

2.1. Study Population

After obtaining institutional review boards' approvals, data from 962 consecutive patients who underwent TBx and SBx between April 2022 and January 2024 were prospectively collected at three European referral centers. All patients signed informed consent for the use of clinical information for clinical studies (coordinator ethics committee protocol number: 0040478). This study was performed according to the Standard for Reporting Diagnostic Accuracy Studies [7].

2.2. MRI and Biopsy Techniques

All prebiopsy MRIs were performed using a 1.5-T or 3-T scanner with a surface coil and consisted of multiplane T1- and T2-weighted imaging, diffusion-weighted imaging (DWI), and dynamic contrast enhancement. Scans were reviewed and scored by experienced radiologists using the PI-RADS v.2 or 2.1 protocols. All MRIs had at least one lesion suspicious for PCa, defined as PI-RADS score ≥ 3. All MRI-targeted prostate biopsies were performed with a transperineal approach under local anesthesia with the Koelis Trinity® (Koelis, Meylan, France) ($n = 746$) or Esaote MyLab™ X9 (Esaote, Genova, Italy) ($n = 216$) fusion imaging system. Expert operators (experience > 500 fusion biopsies) performed or oversaw all the biopsies. A minimum of 2 targeted cores per target were taken, followed by systematic biopsies. SBx adopted a standardized template to sample the posterior region of the prostate, typically with 6 cores per lobe, irrespective of the location of the MRI target.

2.3. Endpoints and Statistical Analyses

The primary endpoint of this study was the added diagnostic value of each biopsy modality, with a side-specific evaluation. For this aim, a per-patient analysis was conducted, considering the lesion with a higher PI-RADS score in the case that multiple targets were reported at MRI. The secondary endpoint was the rate of cancer positivity outside MRI targets at SBx, within the same lobe or contralateral. For this purpose, a post hoc analysis was performed on the 643 patients with a positive biopsy, analyzing the location of MRI targets and the location of positive SBx cores. PCa was considered clinically significant (csPCa) in the case of ISUP grade ≥ 2. Continuous data were reported as medians and interquartile range (IQR) and categorical parameters were shown as counts and percentages. The median test and Fisher exact chi-square test were used when appropriate to compare continuous and categorical variables. To identify predictors of out-field positivity, univariate logistic regression was performed initially to obtain unadjusted odds ratios. Subsequently, all variables were put into a multivariable model to obtain adjusted hazard ratios. Variables of interest for logistic regression were PSA, digital rectal examination (DRE), PSA density (as a binary variable, adopting a cut-off of 0.15), previous negative biopsy status, PI-RADS score, and diameter of MRI target. Statistical significance was set at two-sided $p < 0.05$. Statistical analyses were performed with SPSS version 29.0 (IBM Corp, Armonk, NY, USA).

3. Results

Baseline patient characteristics are shown in Table 1. The patients' median age was 71 (IQR 65–77) and median PSA was 7.0 ng/mL (IQR 5.1–10.2), with a median PSA density of

0.15 (0.09–0.23). Most patients were biopsy-naïve (82%) and had a single MRI target (78%). Targets were scored as 3, 4, and 5 in 21%, 57%, and 22%, respectively, and were more often situated in the posterior (89%) and equatorial (43%) regions. The median number of cores taken was 3 (IQR 3–3) per target and 12 (IQR 12–12) during SBx.

Table 1. Descriptive characteristics.

Variable	Total (n = 962)
Age at biopsy, yr, median (IQR)	71 (65–77)
PSA, ng/mL, median (IQR)	7.0 (5.1–10.2)
PSA density, median (IQR)	0.15 (0.09–0.23)
Suspicious DRE, *n* (%)	281 (29.2)
Biopsy status - Naïve. - Previous negative biopsy.	 794 (82.5) 168 (17.5)
Prostate volume at mpMRI, cc, median (IQR)	48.9 (35.0–65.0)
Number of suspicious lesions, *n* (%) - Single. - Multiple.	 750 (78.0) 212 (22.0)
PI-RADS score of index lesion, n (%) - 3. - 4. - 5.	 202 (20.9) 548 (56.9) 212 (22.2)
Maximum target diameter of index lesion, mm, median (IQR)	10.0 (8.0–15.0)
ADC value of index lesion, median (IQR)	0.7 (0.6–0.8)
Target(s) location, *n* (%) * - Anterior. - Posterior. - Transitional.	 176 (18.3) 615 (88.9) 134 (13.9)
Target(s) location, *n* (%) * - Apex. - Equator. - Base.	 340 (35.3) 412 (42.8) 229 (23.8)
N of cores taken per target at targeted biopsy, median (IQR)	3 (3–3)
N of cores taken at systematic biopsy, median (IQR)	12 (12–12)

Legend: ADC = apparent diffusion coefficient; DRE = digital rectal examination; IQR = interquartile range; mpMRI = multiparametric magnetic resonance imaging; PI-RADS = Prostate Imaging Reporting & Data System * multiple locations allowed per target.

3.1. Added Diagnostic Value of TBx and SBx

The biopsy results are shown in Table 2. The cancer detection rate of TBx + SBx was 65% for all cancers and 55% for csPCa. Taken individually, TBx diagnosed PCa and csPCa in 56% and 50%, respectively, whereas SBx was slightly inferior, with a detection rate of 55% and 45%, respectively ($p < 0.001$). Grades 2 (27%) and 3 (19%) were the most frequent diagnoses. There was a statistically significant difference for csPCa detection in favor of TBx over SBx ($p < 0.001$). TBx was able to detect PCa and csPCa in 100 (10%) and 82 (8%) cases where SBx was negative for PCa and csPCa, respectively ($p < 0.001$). On the other hand, SBx detected PCa and csPCa in 86 (9%) and 54 (6%) cases where TBx was negative for PCa and csPCa, respectively ($p < 0.001$). When TBx was positive, SBx led to an upgrade in the final ISUP score in 46 (5%) cases.

Table 2. Cancer detection rates of targeted and systematic biopsies.

Variable (Cohort N 980)	Targeted Biopsy	Systematic Biopsy	Targeted + Systematic Biopsy
Number of positive cores, median (IQR)	2 (0–3)	2 (0–4)	-
Biopsy positive for PCa, *n* (%)	539 (56.0)	525 (54.6)	625 (64.9)
Biopsy positive for csPCa, *n* (%)	486 (50.5)	433 (45.0)	555 (57.7)
Biopsy highest ISUP grade, *n* (%)			
- 0.	86 (8.9)	100 (10.4)	-
- 1.	53 (5.5)	92 (9.5)	70 (7.3)
- 2.	232 (24.1)	220 (22.8)	261 (27.1)
- 3.	166 (17.2)	133 (13.8)	184 (19.1)
- 4.	57 (5.9)	51 (5.3)	73 (7.6)
- 5.	31 (3.2)	29 (3.0)	37 (3.8)
Biopsy positive for PCa when the other modality is negative, *n* (%)	100 (10.4)	86 (8.9)	-
Biopsy positive for csPCa when the other modality is negative, *n* (%)	82 (8.5)	54 (5.6)	-

Legend: IQR = interquartile range; mpMRI; ISUP = International Society of Urological Pathology; PCa = prostate cancer; csPCa = clinically significant prostate cancers.

3.2. Cancer Positivity Outside MRI Targets at SBx

Among the 625 positive biopsies on TBx + SBx, out-field positivity (outside MRI targets) was found in 213 (33%) cases in the same lobe of the MRI target, and 208 (32%) cases in the contralateral lobe (Figure 1). Focusing only on csPCa, 195 (30%) were diagnosed in the same lobe but outside MRI targets, and 176 (27%) in the contralateral lobe. The results of cancer positivity outside MRI targets with grade distribution are shown in Table 3, together with the regression analyses. Most missed cancers were ISUP 2 (14% and 13% in the ipsilateral and contralateral lobes, respectively). Around 5% of missed cancers were represented by ISUP 4 and 5. Based on the multivariable analysis, predictors of out-field positivity in the same lobe of the target were positive DRE (HR 1.76, 95%CI 1.23–2.51, p 0.002), PSA density $\geq$ 0.15 (HR 1.61, 95%CI 1.21–3.85, p 0.007), and PI-RADS score 5 (HR 2.16, 95%CI 1.21–3.85, p 0.009). The same variables were also predictors of contralateral out-field positivity as follows: positive DRE (HR 1.50, 95%CI 1.03–2.17, p 0.03), PSA density $\geq$ 0.15 (HR 2.20, 95%CI 1.53–3.16, $p < 0.001$), and PI-RADS score 5 (HR 2.04, 95%CI 1.15–3.61, p 0.01).

Table 3. Cancer positivity outside MRI targets at systematic mapping.

Variable (Cohort N 643)	All PCa	csPCa Only
Out-field positivity of SBx in the same lobe, *n* (%)	213 (33.1)	195 (30.3)
- ISUP grade 1.	39 (6.0)	-
- ISUP grade 2.	93 (14.4)	93 (14.4)
- ISUP grade 3.	47 (7.3)	47 (7.3)
- ISUP grade 4.	26 (4.0)	26 (4.0)
- ISUP grade 5.	8 (1.2)	8 (1.2)
- With MRI target(s) positive, *n* (%).	194 (30.2)	162 (25.2)
- With MRI target(s) negative, *n* (%).	19 (2.9)	12 (1.8)
Out-field positivity of SBx in the contralateral lobe, *n* (%)	208 (32.3)	176 (27.4)
- ISUP grade 1.	32 (4.9)	-
- ISUP grade 2.	82 (12.7)	82 (12.7)
- ISUP grade 3.	48 (7.4)	48 (7.4)
- ISUP grade 4.	30 (4.6)	30 (4.6)
- ISUP grade 5.	16 (2.5)	16 (2.5)

Table 3. *Cont.*

Variable (Cohort N 643)		All PCa	csPCa Only
- With MRI target(s) positive, n (%).		179 (27.8)	158 (24.6)
- With MRI target(s) negative, n (%).		29 (4.5)	18 (2.8)
Predictors of out-field positivity in the same lobe			
	Univariate analysis	**Multivariate analysis**	
PSA (ng/mL)	1.00 (0.99–1.00), p 0.66	-	
Positive DRE	2.03 (1.48–2.80), $p < 0.001$	1.76 (1.23–2.51), p 0.002	
PSA density $\geq$ 0.15	1.76 (1.28–2.43), $p < 0.001$	1.61 (1.21–3.85), p 0.007	
Previous negative biopsy	0.73 (0.48–1.12), p 0.15	-	
PI-RADS score - 3. - 4. - 5.	 Ref 1.40 (0.90–2.17), p 0.12 2.61 (1.61–4.24), $p < 0.001$	 Ref 1.50 (0.93–2.40), p 0.09 2.16 (1.21–3.85), p 0.009	
Lesion diameter, mm	1.03 (1.00–1.05), p 0.005	1.00 (0.97–1.03), p 0.94	
Predictors of out-field positivity in the contralateral lobe			
	Univariate analysis	**Multivariate analysis**	
PSA (ng/mL)	1.00 (1.00–1.00), p 0.33	-	
Positive DRE	1.90 (1.37–2.63), $p < 0.001$	1.50 (1.03–2.17), p 0.03	
PSA density $\geq$ 0.15	2.19 (1.57–3.06), $p < 0.001$	2.20 (1.53–3.16), $p < 0.001$	
Previous negative biopsy	0.67 (0.43–1.04), p 0.07	-	
PI-RADS score - 3. - 4. - 5.	 Ref 0.99 (0.65–1.51), p 0.97 2.43 (1.53–3.86), $p < 0.001$	 Ref 0.96 (0.60–1.55), p 0.89 2.04 (1.15–3.61), p 0.01	
Lesion diameter, mm	1.03 (1.01–1.05), p 0.003	1.00 (0.97–1.03), p 0.80	

Legend: DRE = digital rectal examination; IQR = interquartile range; mpMRI; ISUP = International Society of Urological Pathology; PCa = prostate cancer; csPCa = clinically significant prostate cancer; SBx = systematic biopsy.

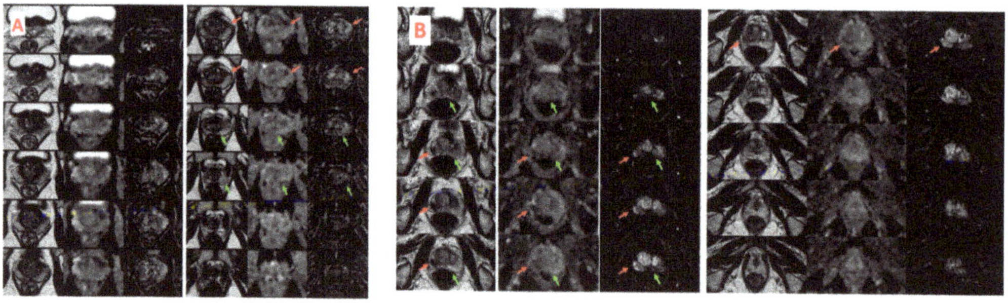

Figure 1. (**A**): *Out-field positivity in the same lobe of the MRI target.* MRI detected a PIRADS 4 lesion (red arrow) in the left anterior peripheral zone at the mid-portion of the prostate. This finding was confirmed by fusion biopsy, which identified ISUP 3 adenocarcinoma in the target area. Additionally, a focus of ISUP 3 adenocarcinoma was found in the left paramedian apical region where the MRI was negative (green arrow). (**B**): *Out-field positivity in the lobe contralateral to the MRI target.* MRI detected a PIRADS 5 lesion in the right peripheral zone in the posterolateral sector of the basal and middle zone (red arrow). Fusion biopsy identified ISUP 5 adenocarcinoma in the target area. Additionally, ISUP 5 adenocarcinoma was also found in the contralateral lobe, in the left peripheral zone at the base in the posteromedial sector, where the MRI (green arrow) showed no significant changes.

4. Discussion

The role achieved by MRI in the diagnostic pathway of PCa is not in question and is supported by strong evidence [1,8]. The PRECISION study demonstrated that MRI-targeted biopsy in men with an MRI-suspicious lesion leads to more significant cancers being identified and fewer insignificant cancers being diagnosed. The European guidelines recommend the execution of systematic mapping after TBx, given the potential presence of mpMRI-invisible csPCa, estimated at 10–20% [9]. However, the diagnostic benefit of SBx has been recently reduced to 5–7% [3,4,10]. In a recent multicentric study, we showed that SBx in addition to TBx improved the detection rate only by 4% for all PCa and by 3% for csPCa [6]. Similar results were found by Cauli et al., who showed an increase of 3% for all PCa and csPCa [11]. Detractors of SBx claim that the performance of SBx is typically overestimated because of test review bias, given that the physician performing systematic mapping is aware of the location of the MRI lesion and somehow targets the lesion even during systematic mapping [12].

The present study is aligned with the recent literature [3,5,6,13] concerning the superiority of TBx over SBx in terms of the detection rate of all PCa and csPCa. Nevertheless, our results showed that both TBx and SBx identify a non-negligible proportion of csPCa when the other modality is negative (10% for TBx, 9% for SBx), in line with the PAIREDCAP study that concluded that combining targeted and systematic biopsy offers the best chances of detecting the cancer [14].

More importantly, in our study, we focused on the rate of cancer positivity found outside MRI targets, even when the MRI target correctly led to a cancer diagnosis. This issue is essential for treatment decision planning, as the presence of csPCa in other regions of the prostate beyond the MRI-visible lesion could lead to abandoning active surveillance or focal treatment or could make it harder to propose a full nerve-sparing surgery, depending on the burden of csPCa. In a series of 1.992 fusion biopsy patients, we previously demonstrated an alarming rate of 57% out-field positivity, of which 58% were clinically significant, even though that study was limited by the lack of data on the precise location of systematic cores [6]. The present study showed that 30% of our patients with a positive biopsy had at least one core of csPCa in the same lobe but outside the MRI target, and—even more alarmingly—27% harbored at least one core of csPCa in the lobe contralateral to the MRI target. Previously, Choi et al. evaluated 185 candidates for hemiablation and found that 123 (66%) of them had bilateral cancer after radical prostatectomy and 73 (39%) had csPCa in MRI-negative lobes [15]. More recently, Gunzel et al. found that 145 out of 736 (20%) patients with unilateral suspicious lesions on MRI were detected with contralateral PCa-positive SBx. Overall, 238 of their patients (25%) showed positive SBx outside of the described PI-RADS lesions [16]. Fletcher et al. evaluated a series of 346 patients with a pre-biopsy MRI and a PI-RADS $\geq$ 3 lesion. When TBx was positive, detection of higher grade csPCa on SBx compared with TBx occurred in only 5% of cases [17]. A retrospective analysis of 2.048 fusion biopsy patients by Brisbane et al. found that 90% of csPCa cores detected by SBx were confined in the so-called "penumbra", within a radius of 10 mm from the nearest lesion. Nevertheless, in 18% of patients, csPCa was diagnosed only by sampling outside the MRI lesion, with the yield decreasing with increasing distance [18]. Bonekamp et al. confirmed these findings, with 18% of csPCa discovered outside mpMRI regions even when a 10 mm security margin was adopted, indicating that prostate MRI has limited ability to completely map all cancer foci within the prostate [19]. Our rates of out-field csPCa positivity are even higher, indicating a contralateral disease in 32% of cases. To better identify patients at risk of cancer outside MRI targets, positive DRE, PSA density $\geq$ 0.15, and PI-RADS 5 score can be used as prognostic variables. PSA density was previously found to be associated with the presence of MRI-negative PCa, together with the black race [20]. Recently, Noujeim et al. evaluated the distance of positive SBx from the index lesion and developed a three-tier prediction model, where the only predictive factors for positive SBx were the PI-RADS score and PSA density [21].

All things considered, the omittance of SBx after MRI-targeted biopsies should be discouraged at present given the risk of missing other csPCa foci within the prostate, which might jeopardize subsequent cancer management. Among the strengths of our study is the prospective and multicentric design. The limitations of our study are the presence of multiple operators, different settings and types of MRIs, different habits in performing SBx, and the absence of central radiological and pathological revision. MRIs were performed in both high- and low-volume centers, and **their** quality was not centrally reviewed, which might have introduced bias. On the other hand, biopsies were performed in referral centers with a high level of expertise.

5. Conclusions

Both TBx and SBx identify a non-negligible proportion of csPCa when the other modality is negative. The performance of SBx after TBx should always be considered given the risk of missing other csPCa foci within the prostate, especially in patients with positive DRE, PSA density $\geq$ 0.15, and PIRADS 5 lesions.

Author Contributions: M.O., R.D.: project development, manuscript writing; A.D., Y.A.S., M.G. and G.A.-D.: data collection; M.O., G.C.: data analysis; G.M., A.P., G.C.: manuscript editing; R.F., P.G.: supervision. All authors have read and agreed to the published version of the manuscript.

Funding: This research received no external funding.

Institutional Review Board Statement: The study was approved by the "A.O.U. Città della Salute e della Scienza" ethics committee as coordinator center (N. 0040478/2020).

Informed Consent Statement: All enrolled patients signed an informed consent before participating in this study.

Data Availability Statement: The data presented in this study are available on request from the corresponding author.

Conflicts of Interest: The authors received no funding for this study. The authors have no competing interests to declare that are relevant to the content of this article.

References

1. Mottet, N.; Cornford, P.; van den Bergh, R.C.N.; Briers, E.; Eberli, D.; De Meerleer, G.; De Santis, M.; Gillessen, S.; Grummet, J.; Henry, A.M.; et al. EAU-EANM-ESTRO-ESUR-ISUP-SIOG-Guidelines-on-Prostate-Cancer-2023_2023-06-13-141145 n.d. Available online: https://d56bochluxqnz.cloudfront.net/documents/pocket-guidelines/EAU-EANM-ESTRO-ESUR-ISUP-SIOG-Pocket-on-Prostate-Cancer-2023.pdf (accessed on 1 July 2024).
2. Drost, F.-J.H.; Osses, D.; Nieboer, D.; Bangma, C.H.; Steyerberg, E.W.; Roobol, M.J.; Schoots, I.G. Prostate Magnetic Resonance Imaging, with or without Magnetic Resonance Imaging-targeted Biopsy, and Systematic Biopsy for Detecting Prostate Cancer: A Cochrane Systematic Review and Meta-analysis. *Eur. Urol.* **2019**, *77*, 78–94. [CrossRef] [PubMed]
3. Rouvière, O.; Puech, P.; Renard-Penna, R.; Claudon, M.; Roy, C.; Mège-Lechevallier, F.; Decaussin-Petrucci, M.; Dubreuil-Chambardel, M.; Magaud, L.; Remontet, L.; et al. Use of prostate systematic and targeted biopsy on the basis of multiparametric MRI in biopsy-naive patients (MRI-FIRST): A prospective, multicentre, paired diagnostic study. *Lancet Oncol.* **2019**, *20*, 100–109. [CrossRef] [PubMed]
4. van der Leest, M.; Cornel, E.; Israël, B.; Hendriks, R.; Padhani, A.R.; Hoogenboom, M.; Zamecnik, P.; Bakker, D.; Setiasti, A.Y.; Veltman, J.; et al. Head-to-head Comparison of Transrectal Ultrasound-guided Prostate Biopsy Versus Multiparametric Prostate Resonance Imaging with Subsequent Magnetic Resonance-guided Biopsy in Biopsy-naïve Men with Elevated Prostate-specific Antigen: A Large Prospective Multicenter Clinical Study. *Eur. Urol.* **2019**, *75*, 570–578. [CrossRef] [PubMed]
5. Bourgeno, H.-A.; Jabbour, T.; Baudewyns, A.; Lefebvre, Y.; Ferriero, M.; Simone, G.; Fourcade, A.; Fournier, G.; Oderda, M.; Gontero, P.; et al. The Added Value of Side-specific Systematic Biopsy in Patients Diagnosed by Magnetic Resonance Imaging–targeted Prostate Biopsy. *Eur. Urol. Oncol.* 2024, *in press*. [CrossRef]
6. Oderda, M.; Albisinni, S.; Benamran, D.; Calleris, G.; Ciccariello, M.; Dematteis, A.; Diamand, R.; Descotes, J.; Fiard, G.; Forte, V.; et al. Accuracy of elastic fusion biopsy: Comparing prostate cancer detection between targeted and systematic biopsy. *Prostate* **2023**, *83*, 162–168. [CrossRef] [PubMed]
7. Bossuyt, P.M.; Reitsma, J.B.; Bruns, D.E.; Gatsonis, C.A.; Glasziou, P.P.; Irwig, L.; Lijmer, J.G.; Moher, D.; Rennie, D.; de Vet, H.C.; et al. STARD 2015: An updated list of essential items for reporting diagnostic accuracy studies. *Clin. Chem.* **2015**, *61*, 1446–1452. [CrossRef] [PubMed]

8. Kasivisvanathan, V.; Rannikko, A.S.; Borghi, M.; Panebianco, V.; Mynderse, L.A.; Vaarala, M.H.; Briganti, A.; Budäus, L.; Hellawell, G.; Hindley, R.G.; et al. MRI-Targeted or Standard Biopsy for Prostate-Cancer Diagnosis. *N. Engl. J. Med.* **2018**, *378*, 1767–1777. [CrossRef] [PubMed]
9. Ahmed, H.U.; El-Shater Bosaily, A.; Brown, L.C.; Gabe, R.; Kaplan, R.; Parmar, M.K.; Collaco-Moraes, Y.; Ward, K.; Hindley, R.G.; Freeman, A.; et al. Diagnostic accuracy of multi-parametric MRI and TRUS biopsy in prostate cancer (PROMIS): A paired validating confirmatory study. *Lancet* **2017**, *389*, 815–822. [CrossRef] [PubMed]
10. Exterkate, L.; Wegelin, O.; Barentsz, J.O.; van der Leest, M.G.; Kummer, J.A.; Vreuls, W.; de Bruin, P.C.; Bosch, J.R.; van Melick, H.H.; Somford, D.M. Is There Still a Need for Repeated Systematic Biopsies in Patients with Previous Negative Biopsies in the Era of Magnetic Resonance Imaging-targeted Biopsies of the Prostate? *Eur. Urol. Oncol.* **2020**, *3*, 216–223. [CrossRef] [PubMed]
11. Cauni, V.; Stanescu, D.; Tanase, F.; Mihai, B.; Persu, C. Magnetic resonance/ultrasound fusion targeted biopsy of the prostate can be improved by adding systematic biopsy. *Med. Ultrason.* **2021**, *23*, 277–282. [CrossRef]
12. Kasivisvanathan, V.; Emberton, M.; Moore, C.M. There Is No Longer a Role for Systematic Biopsies in Prostate Cancer Diagnosis. *Eur. Urol. Open Sci.* **2022**, *38*, 12–13. [CrossRef] [PubMed]
13. Hagens, M.J.; Fernandez Salamanca, M.; Padhani, A.R.; van Leeuwen, P.J.; van der Poel, H.G.; Schoots, I.G. Diagnostic Performance of a Magnetic Resonance Imaging-directed Targeted plus Regional Biopsy Approach in Prostate Cancer Diagnosis: A Systematic Review and Meta-analysis. *Eur. Urol. Open Sci.* **2022**, *40*, 95–103. [CrossRef] [PubMed]
14. Elkhoury, F.F.; Felker, E.R.; Kwan, L.; Sisk, A.E.; Delfin, M.; Natarajan, S.; Marks, L.S. Comparison of Targeted vs. Systematic Prostate Biopsy in Men Who Are Biopsy Naive: The Prospective Assessment of Image Registration in the Diagnosis of Prostate Cancer (PAIREDCAP) Study. *JAMA Surg.* **2019**, *154*, 811–818. [CrossRef] [PubMed]
15. Choi, Y.H.; Yu, J.W.; Kang, M.Y.; Sung, H.H.; Jeong, B.C.; Seo, S.I.; Jeon, S.S.; Lee, H.M.; Jeon, H.G. Combination of multiparametric magnetic resonance imaging and transrectal ultrasound-guided prostate biopsies is not enough for identifying patients eligible for hemiablative focal therapy for prostate cancer. *World J. Urol.* **2019**, *37*, 2129–2135. [CrossRef] [PubMed]
16. Günzel, K.; Magheli, A.; Busch, J.; Baco, E.; Cash, H.; Heinrich, S.; Edler, D.; Schostak, M.; Borgmann, H.; Schlegel, J.; et al. Evaluation of systematic prostate biopsies when performing transperineal MRI/TRUS fusion biopsy with needle tracking—What is the additional value? *Int. Urol. Nephrol.* **2022**, *54*, 2477–2483. [CrossRef] [PubMed]
17. Fletcher, S.A.; Alshak, M.N.; Jing, Y.; Singla, N.; Han, M.; Allaf, M.E.; Pavlovich, C.P. CHARACTERIZING CLINICALLY SIGNIFICANT PROSTATE CANCER DETECTED ONLY BY SYSTEMATIC BIOPSY IN AN MRI-TARGETED BIOPSY PARADIGM. *Urol. Oncol. Semin. Orig. Investig.* **2024**, *42*, S84. [CrossRef]
18. Brisbane, W.G.; Priester, A.M.; Ballon, J.; Kwan, L.; Delfin, M.K.; Felker, E.R.; Sisk, A.E.; Hu, J.C.; Marks, L.S. Targeted Prostate Biopsy: Umbra, Penumbra, and Value of Perilesional Sampling. *Eur. Urol.* **2022**, *82*, 303–310. [CrossRef]
19. Bonekamp, D.; Schelb, P.; Wiesenfarth, M.; Kuder, T.A.; Deister, F.; Stenzinger, A.; Nyarangi-Dix, J.; Röthke, M.; Hohenfellner, M.; Schlemmer, H.-P.; et al. Histopathological to multiparametric MRI spatial mapping of extended systematic sextant and MR/TRUS-fusion-targeted biopsy of the prostate. *Eur. Radiol.* **2019**, *29*, 1820–1830. [CrossRef] [PubMed]
20. Kuhlmann, P.K.; Chen, M.; Luu, M.; Naser-Tavakolian, A.; Patel, D.N.; Kim, H.L.; Saouaf, R.; Daskivich, T.J. Patient- and tumor-level risk factors for MRI-invisible prostate cancer. *Prostate Cancer Prostatic Dis.* **2021**, *24*, 794–801. [CrossRef]
21. Noujeim, J.P.; Belahsen, Y.; Lefebvre, Y.; Lemort, M.; Deforche, M.; Sirtaine, N.; Martin, R.; Roumeguère, T.; Peltier, A.; Diamand, R. Optimizing multiparametric magnetic resonance imaging-targeted biopsy and detection of clinically significant prostate cancer: The role of perilesional sampling. *Prostate Cancer Prostatic Dis.* **2023**, *26*, 575–580. [CrossRef] [PubMed]

Current Oncology MDPI

Article

Quantitative Analysis of Prostate MRI: Correlation between Contrast-Enhanced Magnetic Resonance Fingerprinting and Dynamic Contrast-Enhanced MRI Parameters

Moon-Hyung Choi [1], Young-Joon Lee [1,*], Dongyeob Han [2] and Dong-Hyun Kim [3]

[1] Department of Radiology, Eunpyeong St. Mary's Hospital, College of Medicine, The Catholic University of Korea, Seoul 03312, Republic of Korea; cmh@catholic.ac.kr
[2] Siemens Healthineers Ltd., Seoul 06620, Republic of Korea; dongyeob.han@siemens-healthineers.com
[3] School of Electrical and Electronic Engineering, Yonsei University, Seoul 03722, Republic of Korea; donghyunkim@yonsei.ac.kr
* Correspondence: yjleerad@catholic.ac.kr; Tel.: +82-2-2030-3014

Abstract: This research aimed to assess the relationship between contrast-enhanced (CE) magnetic resonance fingerprinting (MRF) values and dynamic contrast-enhanced (DCE) MRI parameters including (K^{trans}, K_{ep}, V_e, and iAUC). To evaluate the correlation between the MRF-derived values (T1 and T2 values, CE T1 and T2 values, T1 and T2 change) and DCE-MRI parameters and the differences in the parameters between prostate cancer and noncancer lesions in 68 patients, two radiologists independently drew regions-of-interest (ROIs) at the focal prostate lesions. Prostate cancer was identified in 75% (51/68) of patients. The CE T2 value was significantly lower in prostate cancer than in noncancer lesions in the peripheral zone and transition zone. K^{trans}, K_{ep}, and iAUC were significantly higher in prostate cancer than noncancer lesions in the peripheral zone ($p < 0.05$), but not in the transition zone. The CE T1 value was significantly correlated with K^{trans}, V_e, and iAUC in prostate cancer, and the CE T2 value was correlated to V_e in noncancer. Some CE MRF values are different between prostate cancer and noncancer tissues and correlate with DCE-MRI parameters. Prostate cancer and noncancer tissues may have different characteristics regarding contrast enhancement.

Keywords: magnetic resonance fingerprinting; dynamic contrast-enhanced magnetic resonance imaging; quantitative analysis; prostate; prostate neoplasm

1. Introduction

The Prostate Imaging—Reporting and Data System (PI-RADS) recommends a multiparametric prostate MRI protocol that encompasses T2-weighted imaging (T2WI), T1-weighted imaging (T1WI), diffusion-weighted imaging (DWI), and dynamic contrast-enhanced (DCE) MR [1]. As a contrast material and additional scan time are necessary to obtain DCE MRI, the usefulness of biparametric MRI without DEC MRI has been proven [2–4]. However, DCE MRI helps to diagnose clinically significant prostate cancer in the peripheral zone that shows early enhancement, especially in the case where DWI is degraded [5]. PI-RADS recommends qualitatively reviewing DCE MRI and determining whether early enhancement is present in the focal lesion. Although visual analysis based on the relative signal intensity of the lesion compared to the surrounding normal tissue is the common way to interpret DCE MRI, research on quantitative analyses has continued to produce objective parameters [6].

DCE MRI, which repeatedly obtains many images on the same section with a very short time interval, provides a change in signal intensity in the pixel over time. PI-RADS version 1 suggested interpreting DCE MRI by classifying time-intensity curves among three types [7]. Some studies have shown a high proportion of type 3 curves (rapid enhancement and washout) in prostate cancer [8,9]. However, curve type analysis showed poor performance in differentiating prostate cancer from healthy tissue [10]. Moreover, quantitative DCE parameters (K^{trans}, K_{ep}, V_e, and iAUC) from the Tofts model have been suggested to explain the pharmacokinetic characteristics of contrast material in prostate cancer [11]. K^{trans}, K_{ep}, and iAUC are higher in prostate cancer than in benign or normal tissue and are higher in more aggressive cancer than in less aggressive cancer, especially in the peripheral zone [9,12–15].

In terms of quantitative analysis, magnetic resonance fingerprinting (MRF) has emerged as a method to measure multiple tissue properties with relatively shorter scan times than conventional mapping methods [16]. MRF-derived T1 or T2 values were significantly lower in prostate cancer than in noncancer or benign tissue [17–19]. In some research, MRF was acquired before and after contrast enhancement, and the T1 value significantly decreased on contrast-enhanced (CE) MRF compared with nonenhanced (NE) MRF [20]. The contrast-enhanced T1 and T2 values exhibited significant differences when comparing prostate cancer to normal tissue [21]. However, the CE MRF-derived T1 and T2 values of prostate cancer were not explored in the peripheral zone and transition zone separately. Additionally, CE MRF values and DCE parameters, the quantitative parameters related to CE MRI, may be correlated. The purpose of this study was to evaluate the correlation between CE MRF values and DCE-MRI parameters (K^{trans}, K_{ep}, V_e, and iAUC) as well as to validate the difference in the parameters between prostate cancer and noncancer lesions.

2. Materials and Methods

The institutional review board of the hospital approved this study, and the requirement for informed consent was waived owing to its retrospective design.

2.1. Patients

We searched all prostate MRI examinations performed in our institution between January 2020 and March 2021. Among 560 examinations, MRI examinations were excluded according to the following criteria: (1) patients with known prostate cancer including post-treatment or postbiopsy status (n = 203); (2) patients who did not undergo prostate biopsy (n = 198); (3) MRI examinations without MRF (n = 77); (4) patients without suspected prostate cancer (PI-RADS $\geq$ 3) (n = 9); and (5) DCE MRI was not obtained (n = 5). A total of 68 patients who underwent prostate prebiopsy MRI and prostate biopsy for prostate focal lesions were included in this study (Figure 1).

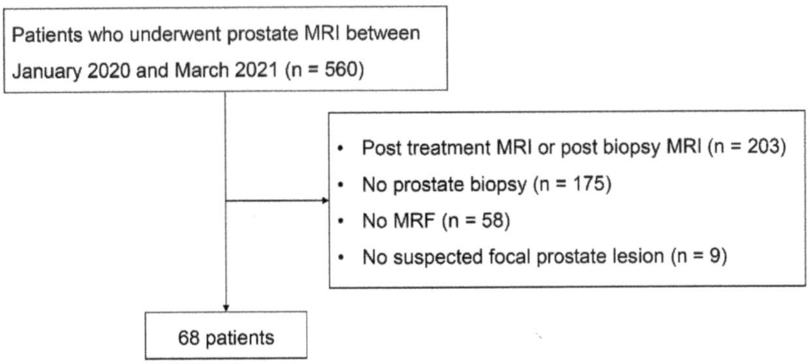

Figure 1. Flowchart of the patient inclusion process.

Patient clinical information, including age and prostate-specific antigen (PSA) level before prostate MRI, was collected. Location and PI-RADS v.2.1 classification were recorded from the MRI reports that were already generated during the clinical process by one of two abdominal/genitourinary radiologists with more than 10 years of experience. If the prostate focal lesion involved both the peripheral zone and the transition zone, the location of the lesion was determined by the center of the lesion. One of the two radiologists performed transrectal ultrasound-guided prostate biopsy using an ultrasound-MRI fusion system (Logiq E10, GE healthcare, Chicago, IL, USA). The radiologist performed targeted and systematic biopsy and reported the location of the targeted biopsy. Pathology results were reported by one of four board-certified pathologists and included the Gleason grade group of prostate cancer, which was defined by the International Society of Urological Pathology, and the number and location of positive cores.

2.2. MRI Protocol

The study involved all patients undergoing multiparametric MRI without an endorectal coil on a 3-T system (Magnetom Vida, Siemens Healthineers, Erlangen, Germany), utilizing a 30-channel body coil along with either a 32-channel or 72-channel spine coil. The specific MRI parameters are detailed in Table 1. Dynamic contrast-enhanced (DCE) MRI was conducted using the Golden-angle RAdial Sparse Parallel (GRASP) technique, with a temporal resolution of 4.3 s for the first 17 s, followed by 7 s for the subsequent 180 s. To calculate the DCE MRI parameters, T1 maps were generated through the variable flip angle technique, employing angles of 2° and 15°. MRF was conducted twice, first before the injection of contrast material and then immediately following the completion of DCE MRI.

MRF has been integrated into the prebiopsy prostate MRI protocol for patients for patients with the clinical suspicion of prostate cancer. MRF data were obtained using a hybrid radial/echo-planar imaging (EPI) trajectory [19]. This involved a golden-angle rotating radial acquisition in the kxy domain, combined with simultaneous EPI acquisition in the slice encoding direction (kz), employing a sinusoidal flip angle to achieve high-resolution MRF data. The scan time of each MRF was 3 min 48 s. For both NE and CE MRF, the same parameters were used: sinusoidal 320 flip angles, TR = 16 ms, TE = 4 ms, resolution = $0.6 \times 0.6 \times 3$ mm^3, FOV = $160 \times 160 \times 72$ mm^3 and scan time = 3 min 48 s. The dictionary was generated based on the Bloch equation in MATLAB (The MathWorks, Natick, MA). The T1 range of the dictionary was 50 msec to 3000 msec with a 10-msec step size and was 3050 msec to 4000 msec with a 50-msec step size. The T2 range of the dictionary was 5 msec to 250 msec with a 1-msec step size, 252 msec to 350 msec with a 2-msec step size, and 355 msec to 400 msec with a 5-msec step size. Dictionary matching using the inner-product method was performed to acquire quantitative T1 and T2 maps from NE and CE MRF.

2.3. Image Analysis

Two radiologists with 10 and 23 years of experience (each having read over 1000 cases) independently analyzed the DCE MRI and MRF images without access to each others' results. We used commercial software (Syngo.via VB70B, Siemens Healthineers) to analyze DCE MRI and open-source software (ITK-SNAP version 3.8.0 [www.itksnap.org [accessed on 30 November 2023]]) to analyze the MRF maps. Four parameters were calculated from the DCE MRI: K^{trans} (volume transfer constant that represents the leakage of contrast from the vascular to the extravascular component); V_e (fractional volume of extravascular extracellular space [EES] per unit tissue volume); K_{ep} (reflux rate constant that describes contrast reflux from the EES back into the vascular component); and the initial area under the time-to-signal intensity curve (iAUC) measured during the first 60 s [22]. T1 and T2 values were acquired from the NE MRF maps, and CE T1 and CE T2 values were acquired from the CE MRF maps. We calculated T1 change (%) and T2 change (%) as [(NE value − CE value)/NE value] × 100.

Table 1. MRI parameters.

	Axial T2WI (TSE)	Coronal T2WI (TSE)	Sagittal T2WI (TSE)	3D T2WI (CS 3D SPACE)	T1WI (TSE)	DWI	MRF	DCE MRI (GRASP)
TR (ms)	2500–3000	2510	4220	1800	500–700	5200–6000	16	4
TE (ms)	103	103	100	104	9	76	4	2
Field of views (mm)	180 × 180	180 × 180	180 × 180	200 × 200	180 × 180	200 × 180	160 × 160	200 × 200
Matrix	320 × 320	640 × 640	640 × 640	577 × 577	320 × 320	120 × 108	256 × 256	224 × 224
Resolution (mm)	0.6 × 0.6	0.3 × 0.3	0.3 × 0.3	0.3 × 0.3	0.6 × 0.6	1.7 × 1.7	0.6 × 0.6	0.9 × 0.9
Flip angle (degrees)	136	136	120	135	120	90	Sinusoidal flip angle	12
Slice thickness (mm)	3	3	3	0.6	3	3	3	3
Gap	0	0	0	0	0	0	0	0
NEX	2	2	6	2	2	2, 2, 9, 9	1	1
B values (s/mm^2)	-	-	-	-	-	0, 100, 1000, 1500	-	-
Acquisition time (min:s)	3:32	3:17	3:17	4:55	3:35	5:58	3:48	3:41

TR, repetition time; TE, echo time; T2WI, T2-weighted image; TSE, Turbo spin echo; CS, compressed sensing; SPACE, sampling perfection with application-optimized contrasts using different flip angle evolution; T1WI, T1-weighted image; DWI, diffusion-weighted image; MRF, magnetic resonance fingerprinting; DCE MRI, dynamic contrast-enhanced MRI; GRASP, Golden-angle RAdial Sparse Parallel MRI; NEX, number of excitations.

Rough information about the location of the most severe prostate focal lesion (right or left, peripheral zone or transition zone) that was reported in the clinical MRI report was provided to the radiologists. However, they were unaware of the biopsy results. They independently drew a region-of-interest (ROI) covering the abnormal focal lesion on the axial image that contained the largest diameter of the lesion. The average values of the parameters were extracted from the ROIs. The images of a representative case are presented in Figure 2.

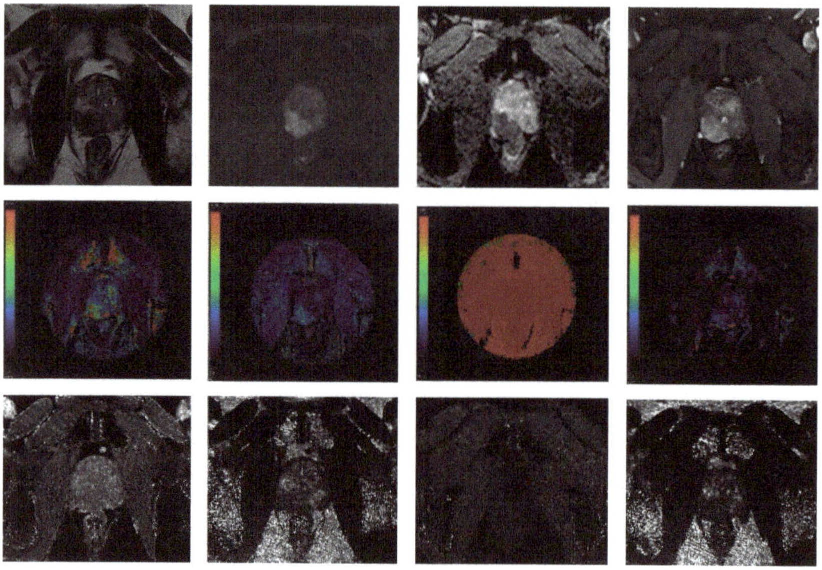

Figure 2. A 66-year-old patient with elevated prostate-specific antigen (15.5 ng/mL).

A 2.5 cm hypointense bulging lesion was detected in the right peripheral zone on the T2-weighted image (T2WI) with a high signal intensity on the B = 1500 mm^2/s diffusion-weighted image (DWI), a low value on the apparent diffusion coefficient (ADC) map, and early enhancement on the dynamic contrast-enhanced (DCE) MRI (T2WI, DWI, ADC map and DCE MRI in order from left, top row). The DCE parametric maps (K^{trans}, K_{ep}, V_e, and iAUC in order, middle row) and MRF maps (nonenhanced [NE] T1, NE T2, contrast-enhanced [CE] T1, and CE T2 maps in order, bottom row) are presented.

2.4. Statistical Analysis

The characteristics of the patients were summarized by presenting the mean and standard deviation for continuous variables, and the frequency and percentage for categorical variables.

Inter-reader agreement for all image parameters was assessed with an intraclass correlation coefficient (ICC). The ICC was interpreted as <0.5, poor; 0.5–0.75, moderate; 0.75–0.9, good; and >0.9, excellent agreement.

Prostate focal lesions were classified into prostate cancer and noncancer according to the biopsy results. We compared the clinical characteristics and quantitative parameters between prostate cancer and noncancer by lesions using Student's *t* tests. The analysis of the correlations between the DCE MRI parameters and MRF values was conducted through Pearson's correlation tests. For statistical analysis, SPSS software version 24.0 (IBM, Armonk, NY, USA) and GraphPad Prism version 8.0 (GraphPad Software, Inc., La Jolla, CA, USA) were used. A p value below 0.05 was regarded as statistically significant.

3. Results

Table 2 shows the characteristics of the patients. The mean PSA of the patients was 37.7 ± 112.2 ng/mL. The prostate focal lesion was located in the peripheral zone in 46 patients (67.6%). More than half of the lesions (51.5%) were classified as PI-RADS 5. Prostate cancer was diagnosed in 51 patients (75.0%), and prostate cancer with Gleason grade group 1 was diagnosed in 4 patients.

Table 2. Baseline characteristics of patients.

Characteristics	Value
Number of patients	68
Age (years)	70.0 ± 10.0
PSA (ng/mL)	37.7 ± 112.2
PI-RADS classification (*n* [%])	
3	1 (1.5)
4	32 (47.1)
5	35 (51.5)
Location of the focal lesion (*n*, [%])	
Peripheral zone	46 (67.6)
Transition zone	22 (32.4)
Prostate cancer (*n*, [%])	51 (75.0)
Peripheral zone	35 (68.6)
Transition zone	16 (31.4)
Gleason grade group (*n*, [%])	
1	4 (5.9)
2	14 (20.6)
3	18 (26.5)
4	10 (14.7)
5	5 (7.4)

PSA, prostate-specific antigen; PI-RADS, Prostate Imaging—Reporting and Data System.

Inter-reader agreement for the CE T1 values and the iAUC was excellent; that for the T2 change was moderate; and that for the rest of the variables was good (Table 3).

Table 3. Inter-reader agreement in MRF and DCE parameters.

Parameters	ICC	*p* Value
MRF		
T1 value (,)	0.825	<0.001
T2 value (ms)	0.898	<0.001
CE T1 value (ms)	0.968	<0.001
CE T2 value (ms)	0.859	<0.001
T1 change (%)	0.892	<0.001
T2 change (%)	0.708	<0.001
DCE MRI		
K^{trans}	0.870	<0.001
K_{ep}	0.854	<0.001
V_e	0.854	<0.001
iAUC	0.904	<0.001

ICC, intraclass correlation coefficient; ADC, apparent diffusion coefficient; MRF, magnetic resonance fingerprinting; CE, contrast-enhanced; DCE MRI, dynamic contrast-enhanced magnetic resonance imaging; iAUC, initial area under the curve.

Patients with prostate cancer were significantly older than patients without prostate cancer (71.8 ± 9.2 versus 64.6 ± 10.8, $p = 0.009$), but the PSA level was not different between the two groups. The PI-RADS classification was higher in prostate cancer (4.63 ± 0.49) than noncancer lesions (4.12 ± 0.49) ($p = 0.001$).

Table 4 shows the differences in the image parameters between noncancer and prostate cancer in the peripheral zone for reader 1 and reader 2. For both readers, the CE T2 values were significantly lower in prostate cancer than in noncancer. The T1 and T2 values were lower in prostate cancer than in noncancer without statistical significance. Among the DCE parameters, K^{trans}, K_{ep}, and iAUC were significantly higher in prostate cancer than in noncancer. In the transition zone, only the CE T2 value was significantly lower in prostate cancer than in noncancer for both readers, although the CE T1 value was significantly higher in prostate cancer than in noncancer by reader 2 (Table 5). No DCE parameter was significantly different between cancer and noncancer.

Table 4. Differences in parameters between cancer and noncancer in peripheral zone.

Parameters	Reader 1 Noncancer (n = 11)	Reader 1 Prostate Cancer (n = 35)	*p* Value	Reader 2 Noncancer (n = 11)	Reader 2 Prostate Cancer (n = 35)	*p* Value
MRF						
T1 value (ms)	1626.1 ± 171.1	1488.2 ± 137.0	0.009	1622.4 ± 169.5	1489.7 ± 210.9	0.064
T2 value (ms)	99.6 ± 27.7	83.1 ± 12.6	0.081	95.17 ± 22.84	79.62 ± 11.70	0.051
CE T1 value (ms)	624.9 ± 77.7	593.3 ± 96.7	0.330	640.1 ± 125.6	608.4 ± 101.2	0.397
CE T2 value (ms)	95.04 ± 26.58	74.9 ± 11.2	0.032	96.41 ± 26.55	71.93 ± 10.51	0.019
T1 change (%)	61.41 ± 4.29	60.0 ± 6.34	0.491	60.76 ± 4.85	58.83 ± 6.79	0.386
T2 change (%)	3.999 ± 8.771	9.424 ± 7.349	0.047	−1.935 ± 16.863	6.904 ± 5.786	0.116
DCE MRI						
K^{trans}	0.209 ± 0.100	0.332 ± 0.101	0.001	0.241 ± 0.104	0.328 ± 0.107	0.021
K_{ep}	0.857 ± 0.382	1.181 ± 0.358	0.013	0.857 ± 0.260	1.146 ± 0.402	0.031
V_e	0.242 ± 0.056	0.298 ± 0.107	0.105	0.279 ± 0.089	0.307 ± 0.122	0.489
iAUC	0.196 ± 0.059	0.301 ± 0.078	0.001	0.227 ± 0.091	0.299 ± 0.084	0.018

ADC, apparent diffusion coefficient; MRF, magnetic resonance fingerprinting; CE, contrast-enhanced; DCE MRI, dynamic contrast-enhanced magnetic resonance imaging; iAUC, initial area under the curve.

Table 5. Differences in parameters between cancer and noncancer in transition zone.

Parameters	Reader 1 Noncancer (n = 6)	Reader 1 Prostate Cancer (n = 16)	*p* Value	Reader 2 Noncancer (n = 6)	Reader 2 Prostate Cancer (n = 16)	*p* Value
MRF						
T1 value (ms)	1596.0 ± 115.1	1575.8 ± 143.7	0.762	1608.9 ± 141.8	1547.9 ± 188.7	0.483
T2 value (ms)	81.77 ± 15.22	76.61 ± 7.93	0.306	76.32 ± 11.44	74.19 ± 9.52	0.662
CE T1 value (ms)	519.87 ± 72.06	591.62 ± 94.44	0.109	490.1 ± 48.8	607.5 ± 103.8	0.016
CE T2 value (ms)	80.32 ± 9.94	70.02 ± 8.13	0.021	72.02 ± 5.56	65.00 ± 7.37	0.048
T1 change (%)	67.15 ± 6.05	62.48 ± 4.67	0.068	69.32 ± 4.29	60.79 ± 4.26	<0.001
T2 change (%)	0.003 ± 14.261	8.629 ± 4.679	0.202	4.107 ± 14.595	12.138 ± 4.957	0.061
DCE MRI						
K^{trans}	0.372 ± 0.165	0.376 ± 0.139	0.954	0.322 ± 0.173	0.384 ± 0.118	0.342
K_{ep}	1.042 ± 0.464	1.247 ± 0.372	0.292	0.998 ± 0.527	1.313 ± 0.420	0.159
V_e	0.356 ± 0.063	0.306 ± 0.079	0.178	0.318 ± 0.055	0.302 ± 0.076	0.650
iAUC	0.320 ± 0.137	0.340 ± 0.116	0.730	0.286 ± 0.154	0.343 ± 0.100	0.317

ADC, apparent diffusion coefficient; MRF, magnetic resonance fingerprinting; CE, contrast-enhanced; DCE MRI, dynamic contrast-enhanced magnetic resonance imaging; iAUC, initial area under the curve.

Correlation coefficients between the MRF parameters and DCE MRI parameters are presented in Figure 3. In prostate cancer, the CE T1 value was negatively correlated, and the T1 change was positively correlated with three DCE parameters (K^{trans}, V_e, and iAUC). The T1 value was not correlated with any DCE parameters. In noncancer, a significant correlation was commonly noted only between the CE T2 value and Ve for both readers. The correlation between the CE T1 value and DCE parameters in the peripheral zone lesions is presented in Figure 4. The CE T1 value was significantly correlated with K^{trans}, V_e, and iAUC in prostate cancer. In contrast, no DCE parameter showed a significant correlation with the CE T1 value in noncancer.

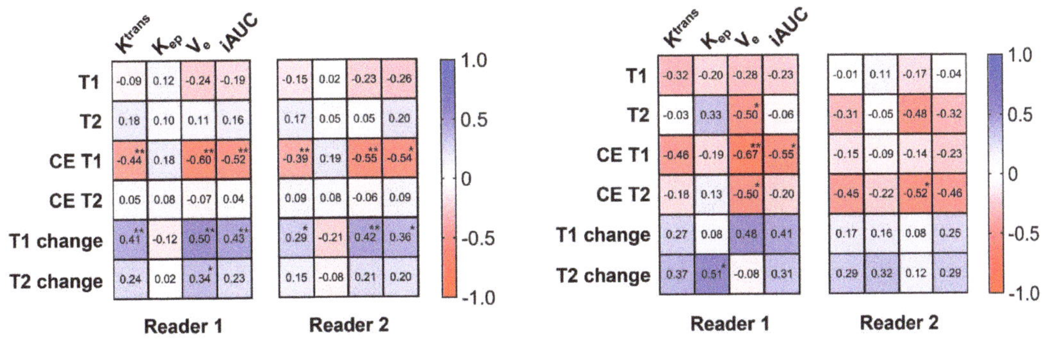

(**a**) (**b**)

Figure 3. Correlation matrix between MR fingerprinting and DCE MRI parameters. Correlation matrices between MR fingerprinting parameters (T1 value, T2 value, CE T1 value, CE T2 value, T1 change, and T2 change) and DCE MRI parameters (K^{trans}, K_{ep}, V_e, and iAUC) are presented for reader 1's result (left) and reader 2's results (right) in cancer (**a**) and noncancer (**b**). * $p < 0.05$, ** $p < 0.01$.

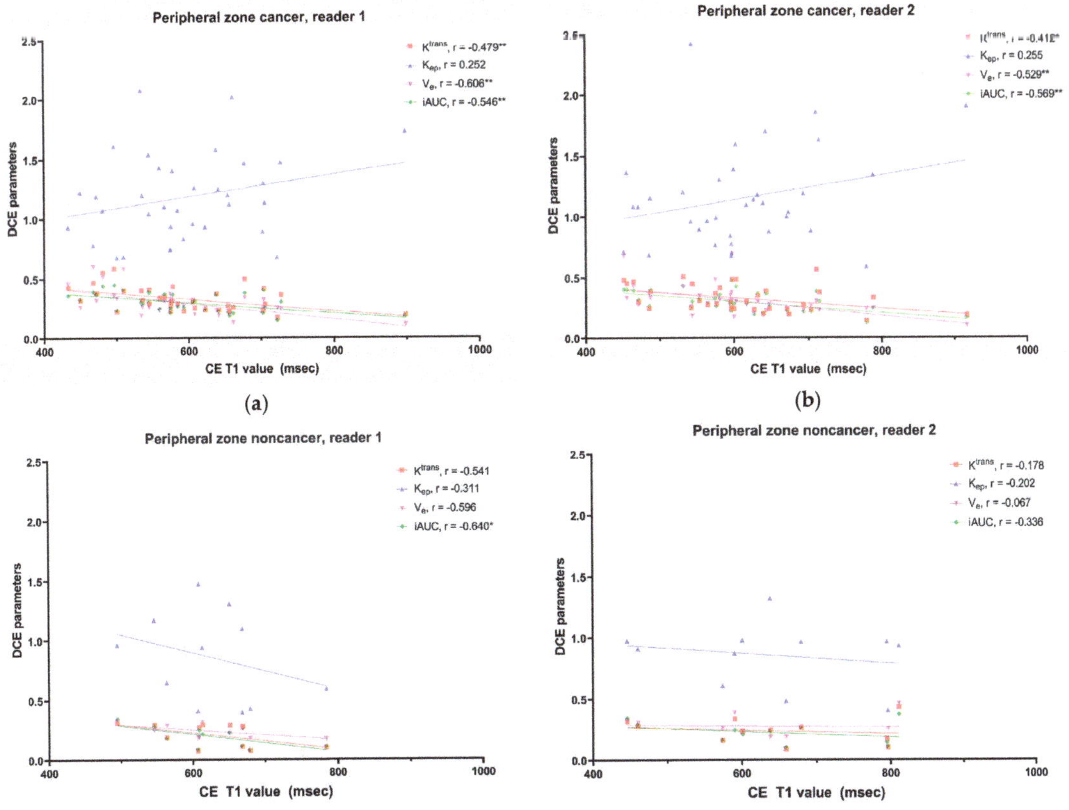

(**a**) (**b**) (**c**) (**d**)

Figure 4. Correlation between CE T1 map and DCE parameters in peripheral zone lesions. Scatter plots show the correlation between the CE T1 value and DCE parameters in prostate cancer and noncancer for reader 1 (**a**,**c**) and reader 2 (**b**,**d**). * $p < 0.05$, ** $p < 0.01$.

4. Discussion

In this study, we acquired NE MRF and CE MRF as well as DCE MRI as a part of prebiopsy prostate MRI in patients who underwent prostate biopsy. We evaluated the parameters from MRF to DCE MRI in prostate focal lesions with PI-RADS classification ≥ 3, and the lesions were divided into prostate cancer and noncancer according to the biopsy results. Therefore, we could evaluate the differences in the MRI parameters between prostate cancer and noncancer lesions in the peripheral zone and the transition zone. Additionally, we investigated the correlations amongst the T1 and T2 values from NE MRF and CE MRF with the DCE MRI parameters in prostate cancer and noncancer lesions.

Among DCE parameters, Ve was not different between prostate cancer and noncancer lesions. K^{trans}, K_{ep}, and iAUC were significantly higher in prostate cancer than in noncancer lesions in the peripheral zone but not in the transition zone. Our study agreed with many studies that showed similar results. A previous study showed that K^{trans}, K_{ep}, and AUC for 90 s after injection were significantly higher in prostate cancer than in the normal peripheral zone or in prostate cancer than in benign lesions [14,23]. Other studies showed that K^{trans} and iAUC were significantly higher in low-grade cancer than in high-grade cancer in the peripheral zone, but not the transition zone [7,13]. No DCE parameter was significantly different between tumor and benign nodules in the transition zone [24]. Ve was not different between prostate cancer and benign tissue or between clinically significant cancer and clinically insignificant cancer in the studies [14,25,26].

We evaluated T1 and T2 values from NE and CE MRF values and the changes in T1 and T2 values. The differences in MRF-derived CE T1 and CE T2 values between prostate focal lesions (including cancer) and the normal peripheral zone or transition zone have been reported previously [20,21]. The differences in CE MRF values between noncancer and prostate cancer have not been evaluated. For both readers, only the CE T2 value was significantly lower in prostate cancer than in noncancer lesions in the peripheral zone and transition zone. As no study has evaluated CE T1 or T2 values between prostate cancer and noncancer, a further evaluation is necessary to validate the results. We interpret this result based on the same context as a previous study; the CE T2 value was significantly lower in prostate cancer than the normal peripheral zone or transition zone [21]. However, the CE T1 value was not significantly different between cancer and noncancer lesions. These results were not expected because we usually use T1WI to evaluate CE MRI. Obtaining CE MRF more than 3 min after contrast injection may be the reason why the CE T1 value was not different between prostate cancer and noncancer. The absolute T1 value of the focal lesion in the delayed phase may not be related to the enhancement pattern in the early phase when prostate cancer commonly shows early enhancement and rapid washout [10,27]. The amount of contrast that is retained in prostate cancer may not be enough to make a significant difference compared to noncancer in the delayed phase.

Regarding NE MRF, both readers' results commonly showed that T1 and T2 values were not different between prostate cancer and noncancer lesions in the peripheral zone and transition zone. Some previous studies showed significantly lower T1 and T2 values in prostate cancer than in noncancer lesions in both the peripheral zone and transition zone [17,18]. In another study that analyzed prostate focal lesions regardless of location, the T2 value was significantly lower in prostate cancer with Gleason grade group ≥ 2 than in noncancer. In the current study, the T2 value of peripheral zone cancer was lower than that of noncancer, but it did not reach statistical significance. Additionally, there was no significant difference in the T1 and T2 values between prostate cancer and noncancer lesions in the transition zone. The differences in the results between the current study and previous studies may be due to the small number of patients in each zone and the noncancer group in this study.

Correlations between CE MRF values and DCE parameters have not been evaluated. The CE T1 value was negatively correlated with K^{trans}, V_e, and iAUC in prostate cancer but not in noncancer lesions. The same results were observed in the peripheral zone. As K^{trans} represents the permeability of the vasculature, a higher K^{trans} means a larger amount of contrast leakage into the EES that causes a greater decrease in the T1 value. Among DCE MRI parameters, V_e showed the strongest correlation with the CE T1 value in prostate cancer. Tissue with a larger V_e, which is the fractional volume of the EES per unit tissue volume, may retain more contrast material, leading to a greater reduction in the T1 value on CE MRF. We noted that K_{ep}, which describes contrast reflux from the EES back into the vascular component, was not correlated with any MRF parameters in prostate cancer and noncancer. CE MRF was acquired after DCE MRI and may represent the characteristics of the tissue in the delayed phase. Therefore, K_{ep} may not affect the CE T1 value in the delayed phase. Thus, this study proved that CE MRF values have different meanings from the DCE parameters; this is understandable because CE MRF values are absolute values measured at a certain time point and DCE parameters are used to measure the pharmacokinetic effects of the contrast material.

There are several limitations in this study. First, this study is a retrospective study. Although all patients underwent MRI-ultrasound fusion biopsy, it was difficult to assure that the focal lesion on prebiopsy MRI was successfully targeted. However, we believe that MRI-ultrasound fusion biopsy is the best clinically available method. Second, the number of patients, especially the number of patients with transition zone lesions, was relatively small. This study evaluated patients who underwent prebiopsy CE MRI, including NE and CE MRF and biopsy. The inclusion criteria for this study were stringent, resulting in a limited number of participants. Despite this constraint on sample size, the findings offer valuable insights. Future research with larger patient cohorts will be pivotal in confirming and enhancing the understanding gained from this study. Third, image analysis was performed on a single axial image that may not reflect the characteristics of the entire lesion. The high inter-reader agreement between the two readers in this study may compensate for the limitation of the single-section image analysis. However, it is noteworthy that despite the high inter-reader agreement between the two readers, the significance of the statistical analyses showed slight variations between them. This could be attributed to the relatively small size of prostate lesions, as including a slightly different number of pixels could lead to minor yet significant alterations in the measurements. Fourth, while statistically significant correlations were identified between MRF-derived values and DCE parameters, these findings did not hold sufficient clinical relevance to routinely substitute DCE-MRI with CE MRF from a quantitative standpoint. Nonetheless, considering that correlations between DCE parameters and MRF values have not been explored previously, presenting these results appears to be meaningful.

5. Conclusions

Some CE MRF values are different between prostate cancer and noncancer tissues and correlated with DCE-MRI parameters. Prostate cancer and noncancer tissues may have different characteristics regarding contrast enhancement.

Author Contributions: Conceptualization, D.-H.K. and Y.-J.L.; methodology, M.-H.C.; software, D.H.; validation, M.-H.C. and Y.-J.L.; formal analysis, M.-H.C.; investigation, M.-H.C.; resources, D.H.; data curation, M.-H.C. and Y.-J.L.; writing—original draft preparation, M.-H.C.; writing—review and editing, M.-H.C., Y.-J.L., D.-H.K. and D.H.; visualization, M.-H.C.; supervision, Y.-J.L.; project administration, Y.-J.L.; funding acquisition, M.-H.C. All authors have read and agreed to the published version of the manuscript.

Funding: This work was supported by the Catholic Medical Center Research Foundation made in the program year 2022, and by the National Research Foundation of Korea (NRF) grant funded by the Korean government (No. NRF-2022R1F1A1069476).

Institutional Review Board Statement: The study was conducted in accordance with the Declaration of Helsinki and approved by the Institutional Review Board of Eunpyeong St. Mary's hospital (PC21RISI0213, 15 December 2021).

Informed Consent Statement: Patient consent was waived due to retrospective study design.

Data Availability Statement: The datasets generated or analyzed during the study are not publicly available due to privacy protection for patients but are available from the corresponding author on reasonable request.

Conflicts of Interest: Dongyeob Han is an employee of Siemens Healthineers, Ltd. Moon Hyung Choi is currently receiving a research grant from Siemens Healthineers, but the research was not related to prostate MRF. The funders had no role in the design of the study; in the collection, analyses, or interpretation of the data; in the writing of the manuscript; or in the decision to publish the results.

References

1. Weinreb, J.C.; Barentsz, J.O.; Choyke, P.L.; Cornud, F.; Haider, M.A.; Macura, K.J.; Margolis, D.; Schnall, M.D.; Shtern, F.; Tempany, C.M.; et al. PI-RADS Prostate Imaging-Reporting and Data System: 2015, Version 2. *Eur. Urol.* **2016**, *69*, 16–40. [CrossRef]
2. Tamada, T.; Kido, A.; Yamamoto, A.; Takeuchi, M.; Miyaji, Y.; Moriya, T.; Sone, T. Comparison of Biparametric and Multiparametric MRI for Clinically Significant Prostate Cancer Detection With PI-RADS Version 2.1. *J. Magn. Reson. Imaging* **2021**, *53*, 283–291. [CrossRef] [PubMed]
3. Kuhl, C.K.; Bruhn, R.; Kramer, N.; Nebelung, S.; Heidenreich, A.; Schrading, S. Abbreviated Biparametric Prostate MR Imaging in Men with Elevated Prostate-specific Antigen. *Radiology* **2017**, *285*, 493–505. [CrossRef] [PubMed]
4. Di Campli, E.; Delli Pizzi, A.; Seccia, B.; Cianci, R.; d'Annibale, M.; Colasante, A.; Cinalli, S.; Castellan, P.; Navarra, R.; Iantorno, R.; et al. Diagnostic accuracy of biparametric vs multiparametric MRI in clinically significant prostate cancer: Comparison between readers with different experience. *Eur. J. Radiol.* **2018**, *101*, 17–23. [CrossRef]
5. Stabile, A.; Giganti, F.; Rosenkrantz, A.B.; Taneja, S.S.; Villeirs, G.; Gill, I.S.; Allen, C.; Emberton, M.; Moore, C.M.; Kasivisvanathan, V. Multiparametric MRI for prostate cancer diagnosis: Current status and future directions. *Nat. Rev. Urol.* **2020**, *17*, 41–61. [CrossRef]
6. Berman, R.M.; Brown, A.M.; Chang, S.D.; Sankineni, S.; Kadakia, M.; Wood, B.J.; Pinto, P.A.; Choyke, P.L.; Turkbey, B. DCE MRI of prostate cancer. *Abdom. Radiol.* **2016**, *41*, 844–853. [CrossRef] [PubMed]
7. Barentsz, J.O.; Richenberg, J.; Clements, R.; Choyke, P.; Verma, S.; Villeirs, G.; Rouviere, O.; Logager, V.; Fütterer, J.J. ESUR prostate MR guidelines 2012. *Eur. Radiol.* **2012**, *22*, 746–757. [CrossRef]
8. Ziayee, F.; Ullrich, T.; Blondin, D.; Irmer, H.; Arsov, C.; Antoch, G.; Quentin, M.; Schimmöller, L. Impact of qualitative, semi-quantitative, and quantitative analyses of dynamic contrast-enhanced magnet resonance imaging on prostate cancer detection. *PLoS ONE* **2021**, *16*, e0249532. [CrossRef]
9. Afshari Mirak, S.; Mohammadian Bajgiran, A.; Sung, K.; Asvadi, N.H.; Markovic, D.; Felker, E.R.; Lu, D.; Sisk, A.; Reiter, R.E.; Raman, S.S. Dynamic contrast-enhanced (DCE) MR imaging: The role of qualitative and quantitative parameters for evaluating prostate tumors stratified by Gleason score and PI-RADS v2. *Abdom. Radiol.* **2020**, *45*, 2225–2234. [CrossRef]
10. Hansford, B.G.; Peng, Y.; Jiang, Y.; Vannier, M.W.; Antic, T.; Thomas, S.; McCann, S.; Oto, A. Dynamic Contrast-enhanced MR Imaging Curve-type Analysis: Is It Helpful in the Differentiation of Prostate Cancer from Healthy Peripheral Zone? *Radiology* **2015**, *275*, 448–457. [CrossRef]
11. Franiel, T.; Hamm, B.; Hricak, H. Dynamic contrast-enhanced magnetic resonance imaging and pharmacokinetic models in prostate cancer. *Eur. Radiol.* **2011**, *21*, 616–626. [CrossRef] [PubMed]
12. Yuan, Q.; Costa, D.N.; Senegas, J.; Xi, Y.; Wiethoff, A.J.; Rofsky, N.M.; Roehrborn, C.; Lenkinski, R.E.; Pedrosa, I. Quantitative diffusion-weighted imaging and dynamic contrast-enhanced characterization of the index lesion with multiparametric MRI in prostate cancer patients. *J. Magn. Reson. Imaging* **2017**, *45*, 908–916. [CrossRef] [PubMed]
13. Vos, E.K.; Litjens, G.J.; Kobus, T.; Hambrock, T.; Hulsbergen-van de Kaa, C.A.; Barentsz, J.O.; Huisman, H.J.; Scheenen, T.W. Assessment of prostate cancer aggressiveness using dynamic contrast-enhanced magnetic resonance imaging at 3 T. *Eur. Urol.* **2013**, *64*, 448–455. [CrossRef] [PubMed]
14. Cho, E.; Chung, D.J.; Yeo, D.M.; Sohn, D.; Son, Y.; Kim, T.; Hahn, S.-T. Optimal cut-off value of perfusion parameters for diagnosing prostate cancer and for assessing aggressiveness associated with Gleason score. *Clin. Imaging* **2015**, *39*, 834–840. [CrossRef] [PubMed]
15. Cristel, G.; Esposito, A.; Damascelli, A.; Briganti, A.; Ambrosi, A.; Brembilla, G.; Brunetti, L.; Antunes, S.; Freschi, M.; Montorsi, F.; et al. Can DCE-MRI reduce the number of PI-RADS v.2 false positive findings? Role of quantitative pharmacokinetic parameters in prostate lesions characterization. *Eur. J. Radiol.* **2019**, *118*, 51–57. [CrossRef] [PubMed]
16. Ma, D.; Gulani, V.; Seiberlich, N.; Liu, K.; Sunshine, J.L.; Duerk, J.L.; Griswold, M.A. Magnetic resonance fingerprinting. *Nature* **2013**, *495*, 187–192. [CrossRef] [PubMed]
17. Panda, A.; O'Connor, G.; Lo, W.C.; Jiang, Y.; Margevicius, S.; Schluchter, M.; Ponsky, L.E.; Gulani, V. Targeted Biopsy Validation of Peripheral Zone Prostate Cancer Characterization With Magnetic Resonance Fingerprinting and Diffusion Mapping. *Investig. Radiol.* **2019**, *54*, 485–493. [CrossRef]
18. Panda, A.; Obmann, V.C.; Lo, W.C.; Margevicius, S.; Jiang, Y.; Schluchter, M.; Patel, I.J.; Nakamoto, D.; Badve, C.; Griswold, M.A.; et al. MR Fingerprinting and ADC Mapping for Characterization of Lesions in the Transition Zone of the Prostate Gland. *Radiology* **2019**, *292*, 685–694. [CrossRef]

19. Han, D.; Choi, M.H.; Lee, Y.J.; Kim, D.H. Feasibility of Novel Three-Dimensional Magnetic Resonance Fingerprinting of the Prostate Gland: Phantom and Clinical Studies. *Korean J. Radiol.* **2021**, *22*, 1332–1340. [CrossRef]
20. Sushentsev, N.; Kaggie, J.D.; Buonincontri, G.; Schulte, R.F.; Graves, M.J.; Gnanapragasam, V.J.; Barrett, T. The effect of gadolinium-based contrast agent administration on magnetic resonance fingerprinting-based T1 relaxometry in patients with prostate cancer. *Sci. Rep.* **2020**, *10*, 20475. [CrossRef]
21. Lee, Y.S.; Choi, M.H.; Lee, Y.J.; Han, D.; Kim, D.H. Magnetic resonance fingerprinting in prostate cancer before and after contrast enhancement. *Br. J. Radiol.* **2022**, *95*, 20210479. [CrossRef] [PubMed]
22. Cuenod, C.A.; Balvay, D. Perfusion and vascular permeability: Basic concepts and measurement in DCE-CT and DCE-MRI. *Diagn. Interv. Imaging* **2013**, *94*, 1187–1204. [CrossRef] [PubMed]
23. Ocak, I.; Bernardo, M.; Metzger, G.; Barrett, T.; Pinto, P.; Albert, P.S.; Choyke, P.L. Dynamic contrast-enhanced MRI of prostate cancer at 3 T: A study of pharmacokinetic parameters. *AJR Am. J. Roentgenol.* **2007**, *189*, 849. [CrossRef] [PubMed]
24. Chesnais, A.L.; Niaf, E.; Bratan, F.; Mege-Lechevallier, F.; Roche, S.; Rabilloud, M.; Colombel, M.; Rouvière, O. Differentiation of transitional zone prostate cancer from benign hyperplasia nodules: Evaluation of discriminant criteria at multiparametric MRI. *Clin. Radiol.* **2013**, *68*, e323–e330. [CrossRef] [PubMed]
25. Oto, A.; Kayhan, A.; Jiang, Y.; Tretiakova, M.; Yang, C.; Antic, T.; Dahi, F.; Shalhav, A.L.; Karczmar, G.; Stadler, W.M.; et al. Prostate cancer: Differentiation of central gland cancer from benign prostatic hyperplasia by using diffusion-weighted and dynamic contrast-enhanced MR imaging. *Radiology* **2010**, *257*, 715–723. [CrossRef] [PubMed]
26. Meyer, H.J.; Wienke, A.; Surov, A. Can dynamic contrast enhanced MRI predict gleason score in prostate cancer? A systematic review and meta analysis. *Urol. Oncol.* **2021**, *39*, 784.e17–784.e25. [CrossRef] [PubMed]
27. Noworolski, S.M.; Henry, R.G.; Vigneron, D.B.; Kurhanewicz, J. Dynamic contrast-enhanced MRI in normal and abnormal prostate tissues as defined by biopsy, MRI, and 3D MRSI. *Magn. Reson. Med.* **2005**, *53*, 249–255. [CrossRef]

MDPI AG
Grosspeteranlage 5
4052 Basel
Switzerland
Tel.: +41 61 683 77 34

Current Oncology Editorial Office
E-mail: curroncol@mdpi.com
www.mdpi.com/journal/curroncol

www.ingramcontent.com/pod-product-compliance
Lightning Source LLC
Chambersburg PA
CBHW062103220926
51850CB00010B/2870
* 9 7 8 3 7 2 5 8 6 0 6 5 4 *